Praise for Ramel Rones...

"Working with Rami for the last five years helped m̲ ̲ ̲ ̲ ̲ ̲ ̲ ̲ ̲ ̲ bilitating back problem, and contributed to a better quality of life. Nevertheless, what has been more important is Rami's consistent teaching of deep breathing and the meditative mind, which has helped me to maintain some calm on the emotional rollercoaster of my life. I believe that stretching, relaxation, and meditation exercises may also have helped me to avoid illness during the long Boston winters. I encourage people to learn and follow Rami's mind/body program."

Larry Lucchino
President and CEO of the Boston Red Sox
March 2006

"Deeply versed, passionate and informed, Mr. Rones is a committed and caring teacher of the Asian mind/body arts, including Qigong, Tai Chi, and Yoga.

This precious exercise shows practitioners how to incorporate positive images from nature into a daily self-healing regimen. The practices come from the oldest traditional teaching, yet offer wonderful antidotes for the accelerated pace of modern life. In learning Mr. Rones' art, novice and adept practitioners alike will find pearls of wisdom."

Ted J. Kaptchuk, OMD
Assistant Professor of Medicine,
Osher Institute, Harvard Medical School
Author of *The Web that Has No Weaver*

"In his twenty years of study with some of the world's great masters of the Asian mind-body arts, Rami received a rare immersion in the inner teaching of Yoga, Tai Chi, Qigong, Meditation, and various martial arts. He has integrated these inner teachings into a powerful balanced mind/body program contained in the *Sunrise Tai Chi* book and DVD.

These exercises are the result of years of testing and refining these deep teachings during Rami's private clinical practice working with students facing life challenges, from maintaining general well-being to surviving cancer. This program is so useful for students at any level of health, whether they are healthy athletes looking to balance their training, or elders who wish to avoid and reverse unnecessary aging.

In *Sunrise Tai Chi*, you will benefit from his clinical experience. He has done the work of determining what works best, and here he has set out an integrated, easy to use set of mind-body practices that allow the student to draw on the best of Eastern meditation and internal bodywork traditions.

In my own experience working with Rami, I have learned so much about how to lead a balanced life while coping with a challenging, potentially life-threatening illness. With Rami's help, and through the exercises he has taught me, I have learned how to energize my life, deal with stress, and stay healthy.

Cathy Kerr, Ph.D.
Instructor, Harvard Medical School

SUNRISE TAI CHI

*In motion, the whole body should be light and agile with all parts of the
body linked as if threaded together.*

The Qi (vital life energy) should be excited,

The Shen (spirit of vitality) should be internally gathered.

Tai Chi Chuan Ching.

— by Zhang, San-Feng

SUNRISE TAI CHI

SIMPLIFIED TAI CHI FOR HEALTH & LONGEVITY

Ramel Rones

with
David Silver

YMAA Publication Center
Boston, Mass. USA

YMAA Publication Center, Inc.
Main Office
4354 Washington Street
Boston, Massachusetts, 02131
1-800-669-8892 • www.ymaa.com • ymaa@aol.com

Editor: Susan Bullowa
Art Direction/Cover Concept: Ramel Rones
Cover Photos and Illustrations: Ilana Rosenberg-Rones
Cover Concept: Vadim Goretsky
Cover Adaption: Axie Breen

ISBN-13: 978-1-59439-083-8
ISBN-10: 1-59439-083-5

10   9   8   7   6   5   4   3   2   1

Publisher's Cataloging in Publication

Rones, Ramel.

Sunrise tai chi : simplified tai chi for health & longevity / Ramel
Rones with David Silver. -- 1st ed. -- Boston, Mass. : YMAA
Publication Center, 2007.

p. ; cm.

ISBN-13: 978-1-59439-083-8
ISBN-10: 1-59439-083-5
Includes bibliographical references and index.

1. Tai chi. 2. Exercise. 3. Health. 4. Longevity. 5. Stress
management. I. Silver, David. II. Title.

GV504 .R66 2007   2007922386
613.7/148--dc22   0705

Disclaimer:
The author and publisher of this material are NOT RESPONSIBLE in any manner whatsoever for
any injury which may occur through reading or following the instructions in this manual.
The activities, physical or otherwise, described in this material may be too strenuous or dangerous
for some people, and the reader(s) should consult a physician before engaging in them.

Printed in Canada.

Table of Contents

Romanization of Chinese Words viii

Foreword by Miriam E. Nelson Ph.D. ix

Acknowledgements xi

How to Use This Book xv

CHAPTER 1: What Is Tai Chi? 1
Introduction 1
History 3

CHAPTER 2: Human Energy: Internal Visualization 7
Goals of the Mind/Body Approach 7
Pillars of the Mind/Body Approach 8
Between Awake & Asleep 12
Physical Movements & Mental Visualizations 14
First Steps in the Journey of Internal Visualization 14
Step 1: Physical Journey 15
Step 2: Mental Journey 16
Step 3: Relaxing the Physical Body 17
Three Spheres 18
Sphere 1: The Lumbar Spine and Abdominal Muscles 18
Sphere 2: The Thoracic Spine and Shoulders/Upper Back/Upper Chest 18
Sphere 3: The Cervical Spine/Top of the Head/Face Muscles 18
Center of Gravity Energy Center 21
Empty & Full Moon 22
Buddhist Breathing 24
Taoist Breathing 24
Pituitary Gland Energy Center Visualization 26
External Baton Visualization 28
Baton Visualization 29
Bubble Visualization (Guardian Energy) 31
Baton/Bubble Breathing Visualization (Bone Marrow-Skin Breathing) 32
Four Gates Breathing 34
Third Eye Pulsing or Spiritual Breathing 36
Baton/Bubble and Four Gates Spiritual Breathing 38

CHAPTER 3: Sunrise Tai Chi Mind/Body Program 41
1. Sitting Meditation 42
2. Standing Meditation 44
3. Cleansing the Body 46
4. Nourishing the Body 47
5. Organ Massage 49

  6. Three Chambers Breathing 51
  7. Vitamin L—Lower Back Stretch 52
  8. Four Gates Breathing 54
  9. Two Bows Breathing 55
 10. Tai Chi Ball 56
 11. Vitamin H—Hamstring Stretch 57
 12. Loosening Leg Joints 58
 13. Loosening the Neck 60
 14. Flamingo Stretch 62
 15. Squat Down 64
 16. Outer Hip 66
 17. Walk and Kick Back 67
 18. Walk Like a Warrior 68
 19. Up Like Smoke, Down Like a Feather 69
 20. Crane Lifts to Heaven 74
 21. Sun Nourishing 75

CHAPTER 4: Understanding Tai Chi Movements 81
Before Beginning Your Moving Stances: Tai Chi Drills & Form 82
    Sacrum Dropped 82
    Head Suspended, Shoulders Dropped 84
    Empty/Full Moon 88
    Elbows Dropped & Sunk 88
    Weight Through the Knees and Not Into the Knees 90
    Turn & Lift Using the Heels 92
    Tai Chi Hand Form 95
Stances 95
    Keypoints about the Stances 96
    Mountain Stance 96
    Begin Tai Chi Stance 97
    Horse Stance 98
    Forward Stance 99
    Back Stance 100
    Empty Stance 101
    Tame the Tiger Stance 103
Moving Stances 104
    1. From Mountain Stance to Begin Tai Chi Stance 105
    2. From Horse Stance to Empty Stance 108
    3. Forward Stance (or Mountain Climbing Stance) to Back Stance 112
    4. From Horse Stance to Tame the Tiger Stance to Empty Stance 114
    5. Forward Stance to Forward Stance 116
    6. From Back Stance to Back Stance 118

Stationary Tai Chi Movements—Drills 120
    1a. Grasp the Sparrow's Tail: Legs Stationary 122
    1b. Grasp the Sparrow's Tail: Legs Moving 125
    2a. Diagonal Flying: Legs Stationary 128
    2b. Diagonal Flying: Legs Moving 130
    3a. Ward Off: Legs Stationary 132
    3b. Ward Off: Legs Moving 134
    4a. Press: Legs Stationary 136
    4b. Press: Legs Moving 138
    5a. Push: Legs Stationary 140
    5b. Push: Legs Moving 142
    6a. Single Whip: Legs Stationary 144
    6b. Single Whip: Legs Moving 144
Ward Off, Rollback, Press, & Push: Legs Stationary 146
Ward Off, Rollback, Press, & Push: Legs Moving 152
The Five Building Blocks 153

CHAPTER 5: Sunrise Tai Chi Form 155
Elements of the Sunrise Tai Chi Form 155
Mountain Stance 156
Begin Tai Chi 158
Grasp the Sparrow's Tail—Right 160
Diagonal Flying 162
Ward Off (Peng) 164
Rollback, Press, and Push 168
    Rollback (Lu) 168
    Press (Ji) 170
    Push (An) 171
    Keypoints 173
Single Whip 174
Cleanse & Close Tai Chi 176

CHAPTER 6: Epilogue 181

Glossary of Chinese Terms 183

Recommended Readings 193

Index 195

Romanization of Chinese Words

This book uses a mixture of both the Wade-Giles and the Pinyin romanization system of Chinese to English. Pinyin is standard in the People's Republic of China, and in several world organizations, including the United Nations. Pinyin, which was introduced in China in the 1950's, replaces the Wade-Giles and Yale systems. In some cases, the more popular spelling of a word may be used for clarity.

Some common conversions:

Pinyin	Also Spelled As	Pronunciation
Qi	Chi	chē
Qigong	Chi Kung	chē kŭng
Qin Na	Chin Na	chǐn nǎ
Jin	Jing	jǐn
Gongfu	Kung Fu	gŏng foo
Taijiquan	Tai Chi Chuan	tī jē chüén

For more information, please refer to *The People's Republic of China: Administrative Atlas*, *The Reform of the Chinese Written Language*, or a contemporary manual of style.

The author and publisher have taken the liberty of not italicizing words of foreign origin in this text. This decision was made to make the text easier to read. Please see the comprehensive glossary for definitions of Chinese words. Both ways of citing Chinese names are used, based mainly on the most common usage for each individual.

Foreword by Miriam E. Nelson Ph.D.

This book by Ramel Rones has been anxiously awaited by professionals and all those dedicated to health promoting activity. We scientists and professionals committed to the dissemination of knowledge which will help people maintain strong and healthy bodies have long needed to refer to a book which clearly makes the connection between exercise and spirit, between the mind and the body. Ramel Rones captures the essence of how the ancient Eastern concepts of mind and body can connect with our modern ideas of health-promoting exercise. He presents this approach in a way that we can understand and begin to use immediately. I have personally worked with Rami and have experienced the benefits and insights of his blend of Tai Chi, yoga, and balance control. This book is a powerful tool for our efforts of motivating people to adopt and use healthy practices to strengthen the body and mind.

I strongly believe that Ramel Rones' instruction of low-impact, stress-reducing exercises and meditations has strong potential to immediately help people that are seeking good quality of life and excellent health and longevity, as well as to complement the journey each individual needs to take with various medical issues.

Some of the medical studies, R-21, which were done with Ramel Rones' approach have showed promising results: improvement in balance, flexibility, and arthritis symptoms, reduction of pain, stress, and anxiety, and improvement in cardio-respiratory function.

Miriam E. Nelson, Ph.D.
School of Nutrition Science & Policy,
Tufts University

Acknowledgements

When I reflect back to understand my journey, I am clear that the people I value and want to acknowledge and thank the most are my father and mother, Arie Rones and Zichria Zakay Rones, for finding me a Tai Chi and Zen teacher to help with the sinus infections and digestive system issues I suffered with throughout my teen-age years. I am grateful for their support and for that of my brother and sister, Gady and Nurit, during the time when I was first learning the eastern arts in Israel, and later, when I traveled at age 21 to Boston in 1983 to study and practice the eastern arts, Kung Fu, Tai Chi, *Qigong*, and Yoga (when everybody else thought that I was crazy and should go to college).

Also, I would like to thank my teacher, or my martial "father"; Doctor Yang Jwing-Ming, first for accepting me into his inner circle of disciples, and secondly for the 23 years of endless teaching. Thank you for teaching me the various eastern arts that have made me so "rich" in knowledge and has given me the satisfaction of being able to help others on both the martial and health levels.

Thank you Master Jou, Tsung-Hwa for being an inspiration on those early mornings at the Tai Chi Farm, and for teaching me the method of tapping into the sun's energy. I would also like to thank my Zen/Tai Chi teacher, Tzvi (Harold) Weisberg, whom I studied with between the ages of 16 and 21. He helped me deal with the various health issues I was experiencing at the time, and just being a teen. Tzvi was able to let go of me and tell me that if I wanted to be more serious I should go and find a better master. I consider him to be enlightened and I hope that I will have the opportunity to spend time with him again.

I also want to thank my Yoga teacher, Patricia Walden, who gave me the tools to understand the soft part, the Yin side, of training and life, and for being a tremendous inspiration to me and my students, by "being Yoga" unlike most people who just train it.

I would like to acknowledge Catherine, Cathy Kerr, superwoman, my student and my colleague in the science world, and her mentor and my friend Ted Kaptchuk. Both have helped bring me into the science world as an equal allowing me to pursue my next challenge, interest, and passion: research. This research will help lead to proving the efficacy of the various principles, techniques, and methodology of the eastern arts in relationship to specific debilitating diseases.

I wish to acknowledge my colleague Dr. Chenchen Wang of Tufts-New England Medical Center who provided the opportunity to design and implement my modified mind-body/Tai Chi approach in her research on treating arthritis of the knee and other joints. Also, I am proud to have had a long relationship with Dr. Miriam Nelson who graciously wrote the Foreword for this book and has been so committed to promoting the importance of strong bodies for good health.

I want to express my love, appreciation and deep respect to my mother-in-law and father-in-law, Civia and Irwin Rosenberg, who are there for me whenever I need it and are not just family, but are my best friends and spiritual inspiration. As Dr. Rosenberg, or Irv, once told me, to help me deal with a major issue in my life, my high expectations, "There are many good men, but there are only a few 'great' men." Irv and Civia are truly "great," and without them my journey would probably have come to a end.

I would also like to say thank you to a few individuals who are my students or have the same interest in putting this knowledge out and have contributed enthusiastically to this project. Thank you Scott Cedeno and Horacio Adrian Duarte for hundreds of hours of transcribing every word I spoke. Thank you Axie Breen for the design work and for helping in so many ways with a positive attitude and a smile. To the YMAA Publication Center staff: thank you Tim Comrie for the beautiful photographs, hard work and patience. Thank you Adison Martin for proofreading. Thank you Susan Bullowa for editing this book. A big thank you to David Silver, who can put on so many hats; first for being such an enthusiastic student, and then for being my DVD director and co-writer, for contributing excellent thoughts and ideas, and for literally putting my knowledge out there. You are doing a great job. Thank you David Ripianzi for your supervision and for believing in me and for the publication of my material. To Leslie Takao thank you for your friendship, proofreading, and other work on this project.

Thank you very much from the bottom of my heart, and from a number of my students, to a small group of individuals I call Sponsors, who believe in my work. They realize that Cancer patients cannot pay to see me every week or even twice a week, sometimes for years. The support from my Sponsors allows me to work with certain individuals without charge, and to have the time to put my knowledge into books and DVDs. Thank you very much to my Sponsors Zichria Zakay Rones, Irwin & Civia Rosenberg, Billy & Meredith Star, Stacey & Larry Lucchino, Judy & Douglas Krupp, and Bertha Kao & Brian Avery.

Last but not least, my lover, partner, and wife Ilana. First, thank you for all the illustrations, drawings, photographs, proofreading, spelling, and grammar corrections. Thank you for always being there for me and with a positive, relaxed attitude. How many individuals can do that? Thank you, my love, for being the best mother for our gorgeous three boys; Stav, Yahm, and Gahl and our new beautiful princess daughter Danielle, and especially thank you for showing me that love does not diminish, but can actually grow, grow, and grow. Isn't life exciting?

—Ramel Rones (Rami), March 2007

David Silver wishes to extend my deepest gratitude to my friend and mentor, Ramel Rones for the opportunity to work together on this and various other projects. Ocean, my wife and partner, my best friend, and my everything—thank you for always seeing the truth. Elizabeth Coyle and Jeffrey Nelson. David Ripianzi and all my friends at YMAA Publication Center. Thank you to all the above, and to my family and friends; you are all my teachers. Special thanks to Master Yang, Jwing-Ming for his limitless teaching and guidance; without you, none of this would be possible.

—David Silver, January 2007

How to Use This Book

In order to obtain the full benefits of this book, first read through it completely to understand the theory and become familiar with what I call the different "mind/body prescriptions," the exercises/visualizations.

Once you begin training, start practicing the physical skills separately from the mental visualizations. Practice the various physical and mental skills individually until you sense that it is time to put them together. Use my concept of the "Art of Using 80 Percent of your Effort" when advancing through the physical skills, which will help you to prevent injuries, leaving the other 20 percent of your attention for focusing on the breath and the mental tasks. Being able to visualize three or four visualizations at once is not easy. It is a process that takes time. Do not overload your brain; give yourself enough time and slack, and do not be hard on yourself.

For beginners, it is natural, when you are trying to put your mind in the energy centers, for other thoughts to steal your mind away from staying focused on the visualization. Instead of fighting your thoughts and trying to pull them back into your energy centers, try to loop them back in a natural, curving arc. Let the thoughts happen and then just loop them back in, and regain your focus on your breath and the sensation of the energy center. When you realize a thought has taken your attention, you can visualize looping your attention in through the Third Eye, into the pituitary gland area or energy center, and connect into the baton in the center of your body, and then lead it down into the lower energy center in your abdomen, your center of gravity energy center. As you read this book, all of these concepts are explained.

Again, this will take time and energy. Therefore, you must invest the time and the effort to achieve these internal goals. Once you achieve them, you can gradually mix this skill with any other stretches, stances, moving Tai Chi drills, and the Tai Chi form we will show you in this book.

Advance through the theory as well as through the action while referring back to the detailed instructions until you have a strong understanding of the various mind/body prescriptions, the separate Tai Chi movements, and the Tai Chi form. Practice the Tai Chi drills and the form both ways, to the left and right. Remember, one of the main objectives of the exercises in this book is to free your skeleton from being a prisoner of the soft tissue. If you cannot perform certain physical skills, it is often because the soft tissue is shortened from lack of use or insufficient stretching. It is restricting the full range of motion of your skeleton. Once you are free of this shortness in the soft tissue, and you have built enough strength, you can do what your body is potentially designed to do and the quality of your life will change tremendously.

Try to experience simultaneously the heavy force from your body's Center of Gravity Energy Center downward, and the light force from the Center of Gravity area upward, and then through the center of the body and the spine. One day you will be able to differentiate between the two at all times. You will discover that when you inhale, it enhances the feeling of the light force through the spine, and when you exhale, you lead the heavy force through the legs.

As you become more advanced or experienced, you will see that you can change this at will. When you inhale, you can emphasize the heavy force through the legs while monitoring the light force through the spine and when you exhale, emphasize the light force through the spine while monitoring the heavy force through the legs. This skill can be very useful in your Tai Chi practice and in developing a stronger ability to monitor your body's internal properties.

Connecting with the forces of nature, especially the sun, is very important. You will need to remember the experiences and sensations which you have had with each one of these natural forces and try to apply them when you are visualizing the forces.

For example, when you "work" with the earth energy, you may recall the experience of working in the garden, digging into the earth with your hands, planting, and feeling the earth between your fingers. This physical feedback can help you have a stronger sensation of earth energy in your visualization.

In the Eastern arts, there is an exercise called Embrace the Tree in which you literally go and hug a tree, or you can emulate this. Recalling a walk through the forest or a time you may have climbed a tree can help you to feel a strong connection to the trees and their energy, which you can apply later in your practice.

When you hike through the mountains, you can sense a connection to them, especially when you stand on the summit and look at the view of the landscape, across a mountain range. You can utilize this powerful feeling in your practice.

If you ever flew in a plane, or if you ever skydived, or perhaps stared at clouds when you were a child, you can have a stronger sensation of the sky when "drawing in" sky energy. If you were an astronaut, you would probably have a stronger sensation of the universe, and the stars!

The bottom line is that you want to connect not just with your imagination, but also with your emotions and most importantly, with your spirit. For example, the mind/body prescription "Walk Like a Warrior" should not only be physical. I want you to add your spirit and literally sense as if you were running through a battlefield to save your family and your country, or whatever it takes to evoke your spirituality. Of course, on the physical level, this walking is an excellent cardiovascular exercise and helps in losing weight. On a spiritual level, your eyes are those of a warrior. The feeling in your entire body is like a warrior. Then once you finish the exercise, you are in peacetime. No more warrior and no more war. Return to your meditative state, with brainwaves between awake and asleep, and with a high spiritual sensation. This skill of changing your energy so dramatically can be very helpful in daily life, in relationships, and in your ability to adapt, to accept sudden changes, and even maybe one day to enlighten.

This journey is not easy. There are obstacles. It takes training, time and effort, and consistent repetition of both the mental and the physical exercises. Eventually you will be able to be like a conductor, able to monitor the many skills at once. By following these guidelines, your results and benefits will be much stronger and they will lead you step-by-step, if not to enlightenment, then to better health and a higher quality of life.

CHAPTER 1
What Is Tai Chi?

INTRODUCTION

Each day, millions of men and women worldwide practice the Chinese martial art Tai Chi Chuan (taijiquan), which has been known for centuries to promote deep relaxation, excellent health, and to prevent injuries and illness. This gentle moving meditation teaches you to find balance between strength and flexibility, increases bone density, while involving all of the various soft tissues in your body: muscles, tendons, ligaments, fasciae, and skin.

Commonly known by its abbreviated name, Tai Chi (taiji) practice improves the circulation of blood and *Qi* (energy), which enhances the body's natural healing capabilities. In addition to learning fundamental Tai Chi stances and postures, these body-conditioning exercises also help you to increase muscle mass and bone density, while the gentle movements continually massage your internal organs, leading to increased flow of blood and oxygen through every cell in our body. Tai Chi is an excellent way to improve your quality of life and daily physical performance quickly. You will learn to relax your body and mind, optimize your internal energy use, and allow the energy from your surroundings to be absorbed into your body and boost your energy system to abundant levels. Relaxation is an essential key to successful practice, and should be the primary goal of students new to Tai Chi.

Each of the movements taught here can be done seated as well, for those who have difficulty or are unable to stand, and for those interested in refining the training by first isolating the upper part of the body. Training on the edge of a chair offers many benefits for beginners and for more advanced students, because it restricts movement, and causes the practitioner to focus on fine-tuning certain aspects, or skills, that are needed in each one of the five building blocks: Body, Breath, Mind, Energy, and Spirit. For example, you will learn to focus on an aspect of the movement, such as turning the waist, and on using certain breathing techniques.

Practiced to both the left and right, this simplified short Yang-style Tai Chi Chuan sequence is a perfect way to balance your practice before moving on to more complex Tai Chi forms, such as the 24-posture form, or the older, long form of 108 postures.

Finally, the "internal" aspect of each movement will allow you to experience the connection between your body, mind, and spirit. This will help you find harmony within yourself, as well as harmony between Human Energy, Earth Energy, and Universal Energy. In the Tai Chi Classics it is written that Tai Chi is originated from Wu Chi and is the mother of Yin and Yang (see symbols below).

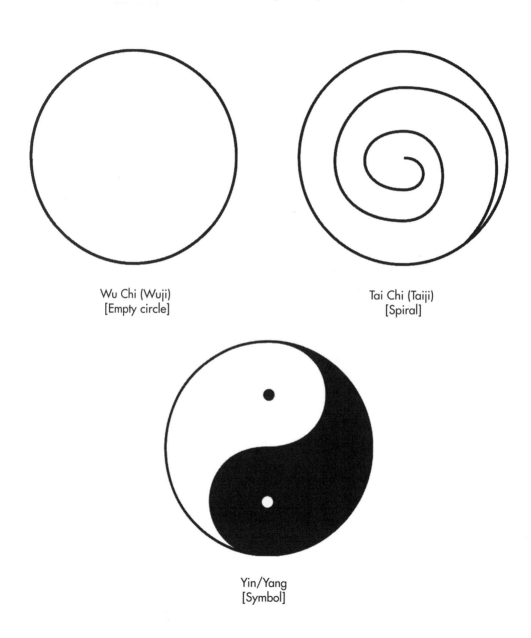

Wu Chi (Wuji)
[Empty circle]

Tai Chi (Taiji)
[Spiral]

Yin/Yang
[Symbol]

HISTORY

Tai Chi, or taiji, is an ancient Chinese philosophy that dates back at least 5,000 years. Some recent archaeological findings suggest that the *Yin-Yang* concept may be over 10,000 years old. *Yin-Yang* theory is based on the idea that everything in the universe is created, developed, and constantly changing due to the interaction, balance, and imbalance of *Yin* and *Yang*, which can be described as any two opposing forces, such as light/dark, cold/hot, or force/yielding. This concept of constant change and *Yin-Yang* balance is an approach to understand the laws of nature, and the universe itself.

Tai Chi (taiji), which translates as Grand Ultimate, is the creative force that lies between *Wuji*, the state of No Extremity, and *Yin-Yang*, the state of Discrimination. In Tai Chi Chuan (taijiquan), this creative force is the mind, the origin of all movement, and therefore the origin of all *Yin-Yang* in the body. This Tai Chi philosophy was later blended with several ancient physical exercises and martial arts forms to create a new martial art style known as Tai Chi Chuan, or Grand Ultimate Fist. Tai Chi Chuan is often shortened to Tai Chi, but the practitioner should be clear about the distinction between the martial art of Tai Chi Chuan, and the more ancient Tai Chi philosophy.

Lao Tzu, an older contemporary of Confucius, wrote and taught Taoist (Daoist) philosophy in the province of Hunan in the 6th century B.C. His classic book the *Tao Te Ching* (*Dao De Jing*), or *The Way of Virtue*, offers insightful discussions of Taoist philosophies which lie in the heart of Tai Chi Chuan.

The essential principles of Tai Chi Chuan can be traced back thousands of years to ancient Chinese health exercises and to Classical Yoga in India. In the 4th century B.C., the Life-Nourishing Techniques (*Yangshenfa*) were being practiced. These ancient exercises included bending, expanding, condensing, and extending movements, breathing techniques, and *Qi* circulation methods similar to the later internal aspects of Tai Chi.

Ancient exercises and breathing techniques, known as *Dao Yin* and *Tu Na*, were created to adjust the imbalance of *Qi* energy in the body, to build more energy, and to increase adaptability to the natural changes in the environment. *Dao Yin* is the art of guiding the energy in the pathways of the body to achieve harmony, and of stretching the body to "massage" the *Qi* pathways in order to reduce *Qi* energy stagnation and to attain flexibility. *Tu Na* is the art of breathing, which was taught and studied in the Buddhist Shaolin and Wudang monasteries.

Other patterns practiced since the Chinese Tang dynasty (600 A.D.), such as Long Fist, Little Nine Heavens, and Five Animal Sports are attributed to the development of Tai Chi. In 800 A.D., a philosopher named Hsu, Hsuan-P'ing developed a long *Kung Fu* of 37 forms. Of these, certain postures still survive in the contemporary Tai Chi form, including:

- Play the Guitar
- Single Whip
- Step Up to Seven Stars
- Jade Lady Works the Shuttles
- High Pat on Horse
- White Crane (originally Phoenix) Flaps Its Wings

Many stories tell of the origin of Tai Chi Chuan, but the most popular legend is that of Zhang, San-Feng, a Taoist (Daoist) immortal and Shaolin martial artist. Zhang is described as an eccentric hermit with extraordinary powers, who died once and was reborn, and whose life spanned a period of at least 300 years, though no one is sure exactly when he lived. According to the legend, Zhang, a monk of the Wudang monastery, created Tai Chi Chuan after witnessing a battle between a crane and a snake. Wudang (Wu Tang) or Wudang Shan, refers to a region in China which includes seventy-two different mountains.

Intrigued by the yielding, smooth evasion, and darting counterattacks of both animals, Zhang's insight in the practice of martial arts are expressed according to four basic principles:

- Use calm against action.
- Soft against hard.
- Slow against fast.
- Single against a group.

He stressed the "internal" aspects of the exercises, and he is credited with creating the fundamental Thirteen Postures of Tai Chi that correspond to the eight basic trigrams of the *I Ching* and the five elements. The eight postures or doors are

1. *Peng*–Ward-off
2. *Lu*–Rollback
3. *Ji*–Press/squeeze
4. *An*–Push

5. *Cai*–Pull/pluck
6. *Lie*–Rend/split
7. *Zhou*–Elbow (striking or neutralizing)
8. *Kao*–Bump (shoulder, hip, knee)

The five attitudes or steppings refer to the five strategic directional movements. They are:

1. Advance (step forward)–*Jin Bu*
2. Retreat (step back)–*Tui Bu*
3. Look left–*Zuo Gu*
4. Gaze right–*You Pan*
5. Firm the center (central equilibrium)–*Zhong Ding*

Tai Chi Chuan stresses suppleness and elasticity and is opposed to hardness and force. It incorporates philosophy, physiology, psychology, geometry, and the laws of dynamics. It promotes highly raised awareness of self and surroundings, both physical and mental.

More recent history with reliable historical documentation traces the lineage of modern-day Tai Chi Chuan back to the Chen family village, Chenjiagou. This style was founded by the legendary Chen, Bu. The Chen family kept its Tai Chi Chuan a secret for fourteen generations. It was forbidden for anyone to teach it outside the family or to anyone untrustworthy. During the early eighteenth century, a young martial artist named Yang, Lu-Chan with stomach problems studied Tai Chi with Chen, Chang-Xing to help heal his ailment. Studying for several years while working as a servant in the Chen household, Yang deciphered many of the secret fighting aspects of the Chen style Tai Chi Chuan. One night, Yang, Lu-Chan was discovered practicing in secret and Master Chen was so impressed by Yang's enthusiasm and level of fighting skill that he broke a four hundred year tradition by accepting Yang as a student. This relationship lasted 18 years until Yang returned to his hometown to teach where he became known as Yan Wu Di—the man who cannot be defeated.

Yang, Pan-Hou (1837–1892) was the eldest son of Yang, Lu-Chan and the teacher of Wu, Quan-You, who went on to create Wu Style Tai Chi. He developed the advanced, small-circle Tai Chi Chuan form which emphasizes the rotation of the waist, coiling of the body, and the development of *Qi* and Spirit. The form of Yang, *Pan-Hou* is the lineage from which the short Sunrise Tai Chi form was derived.

There are five major styles of Tai Chi Chuan, and many lesser-known styles, each named after the Chinese family or teacher that passed it on, in order of antiquity:

• Chen style (陳氏)
• Yang style (楊氏)
• Wu or Wu/Hao style of Wu, Yu-Hsiang (武氏)
• Wu style of Wu, Ch'uan—Yu and Wu, Chien—Ch'uan (吳氏)
• Sun style (孫氏)

Today, Yang style is most popular worldwide, followed by Wu, Chen, Sun, and Wu/Hao.

In Tai Chi combat, if one uses hardness to resist force then both sides may be injured to some degree. Such injury, according to Tai Chi theory, is a natural consequence of meeting force with force, known as "double-weighting." Instead, Tai Chi students are taught to meet incoming force with softness and to "stick" to it, "adhering" to the attacking limb or force and following its motion by remaining in subtle physical contact until the incoming force of attack exhausts itself or can be safely lead and redirected. Achieving balance between *Yin* and *Yang* is a primary goal of Tai Chi Chuan, in your interactions, and within yourself.

As Lao Tzu said in the *Tao Te Ching* over 2,500 years ago, "The soft and the pliable will defeat the hard and strong."

Though the major traditional styles of Tai Chi have forms that differ somewhat on the surface, especially depending upon the performer, there are many obvious similarities, especially in the internal principles, which point to their common origin. Unfortunately, a thorough understanding of the internal aspects of Tai Chi, the energetic circulatory system, and the martial applications, have not been passed down by teachers to many students over the last century, and these important subjects are not commonly practiced in Tai Chi society today.

Of course, Tai Chi can be an excellent health regimen for today's busy lifestyle. The slow, repetitive practice of Tai Chi gently increases and opens the internal circulation (breath, body heat, blood, peristalsis, metabolism, *Qi* energy, etc.). As you progress in the training, this enhancement develops a lasting effect, reversing the physical effects of stress on the body, improving physical health and longevity, and allowing abundant *Qi* energy to be stored and circulated in the body. This repetition also feeds the body's memory, or reflexes, which is stored in the spine, eventually leading to perfectly-tuned body mechanics, alignment, and posture during the Tai Chi form, and at all other times during the day.

CHAPTER 2
Human Energy: Internal Visualization

The existence of *Qi* energy is still disputed in the West, even though this life force has been studied in the growing field of bioelectricity research since the 1960s. However, practitioners of Tai Chi, *Qigong,* and other internal arts do not wait for science to verify the existence of *Qi*. Instead, we train and develop our awareness of this energy in order to harness it for health and martial arts (Figures 1 and 2). For the sake of our health, longevity, and martial arts training, we cannot afford to wait for science to catch up with thousands of years of human experience.

Tapping into the sun, or into other sources of external energy, in order to boost our human energetic system on a daily basis, is a technique that has commonly been used by various Eastern philosophies, including *Qigong* and Tai Chi. Each individual needs to embark on their own internal mind, body, and spirit journey so they can understand, develop, fine-tune, and balance our five building blocks: Body, Breath, Mind, Energy, and Spirit. At the same time, one must progress to the next level and learn to harmonize with the three forces: Heaven, Human, and Earth (Figure 3). This journey is a life-long process, and the rewards are immeasurable, and worth every hour that you spend training, both for health and martial arts (Figure 4).

PILLARS OF THE MIND/BODY APPROACH

Body: Strive to attain its maximum physical potential to create the "best environment" for all systems to function to their fullest.

Mind: Recognize what is viewed in the east as two minds; the emotional (or monkey) mind and the wisdom (or horse) mind. As it is said, "Seize the Ape, Obtain the Horse."

Breathing: Referred to as a tool, or a banana, to capture the monkey mind.

Spirit: Raise and cool it as needed.

Energy: Product of the other building blocks being regulated, balanced, and in harmony with each other and the forces around them.

GOALS OF THE MIND/BODY APPROACH
- Complement Western Treatment
- Develop Sensitivity and Awareness
- Journeying into the Self
- Dealing with and Preventing Illnesses and their Symptoms
- Prevent Disability and Increase Physical Performance
- Empower individuals, families, physicians to play an active role in health care
- Improve Martial Skills

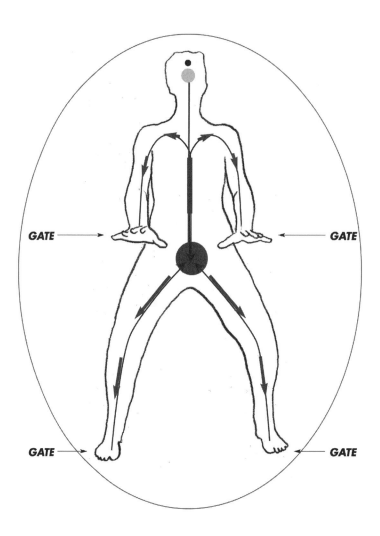

Figure 1. Entire Energetic System I: Baton/Four Gates/Bubble/Spirit

The path of this journey is clear and simple, yet it is difficult to master. Knowing the two secrets to achieving success will make your journey easier and more enjoyable. The first secret is finding a knowledgeable teacher. There is a saying, "It can take you ten years to become a master, but it may take you twenty years to find the right one." Without a teacher, your training will take much longer, and the accomplishment may not be at a very high level. The second secret to success is known by all, but achieved by few: practice, practice, practice.

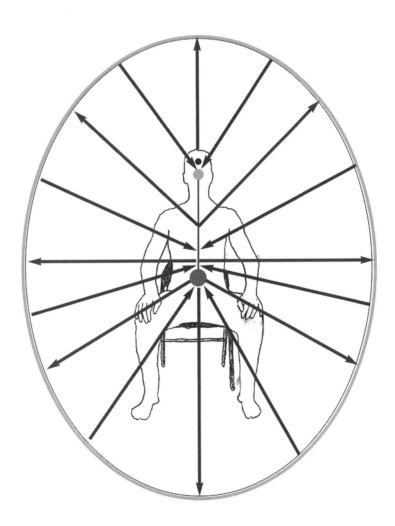

Figure 2. Entire Energetic System II: Baton/Bubble/Spirit

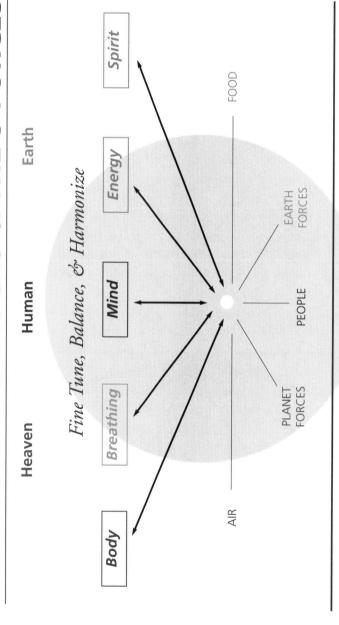

Figure 3.

THE EASTERN ARTS

Chi Kung	**Tai Chi**	**Kung Fu**	**Yoga**	**Meditation**
Science of Energy	Grand Ultimate	Time & Study	Union	Mastering the Mind

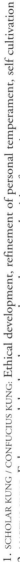

Spirit

*A
Way of Life*

Body   *Mind*

1. SCHOLAR KUNG / CONFUCIUS KUNG: Ethical development, refinement of personal temperament, self cultivation
2. MARTIAL KUNG: Enhance and develop the strength, endurance and spirit of a warrior
3. MEDICAL KUNG: Improves quality of life, complements ongoing western treatment, relieves symptoms of illness
4. RELIGIOUS KUNG: Divided into two categories:
   Taoist - Cultivation of physical body and spirit, merging with nature to achieve longevity and immortality
   Buddhist - Spiritual Cultivation as a way to reach enlightenment, freedom from the cycle of life and death

Figure 4.

BETWEEN AWAKE & ASLEEP

Most Eastern arts seek ways for the practitioner to spend more time in a deeply relaxed state, that is, with a meditative mind. This deep level of meditation is an essential step for achievement in all Eastern disciplines: seeking enlightenment (meditation), better performance (*Kung Fu*), higher quality of life (Taoism), and better health (*Qigong*). Through centuries of accumulated experience, the Eastern arts discovered that the mind is usually in an active state, even during sleep. This has been scientifically researched and verified in modern times. A common realization is that in order to achieve a deep level of relaxation and high skill in internal arts, one needs to develop a concentrated and meditative mind, which can be difficult to reach for any person. In fact, achieving this skill is an art in itself, which has been explored by many disciplines, if not all, such as Buddhism, Zen, Yoga, martial arts, dance, and various sports. Individuals have discovered that by isolating themselves, such as in a monastery or cave, while limiting the food intake and external stimulus, one may create a better environment for the mind and the spirit to remain for longer periods of time in this meditative state.

One enters this state when the brainwave activity slows from the usual beta and alpha brainwaves of daily activity to the borderline near-sleep state between theta and delta brainwaves, which have greater amplitude and slower frequency (Figure 5). Staying aware, and keeping the mind centered and focused in this state is not only difficult, but rare. It is hard to find opportunities in our normal daily routines to spend

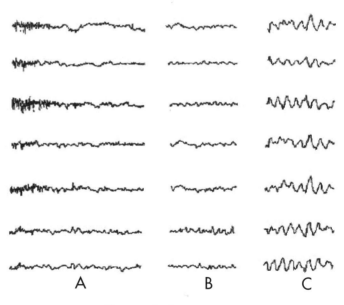

Figure 5. Brainwave patterns

A: Beta brain waves (13-22 cycles). Normal waking state. The pattern changes as abdominal breathing and the relaxation practice begins.

B: Alpha brain waves (8-12 cycles). This state reflects the Relaxation Response, a calm peaceful state of mind with many physical benefits.

C: Theta brain waves (4-7 cycles). Deeply relaxed state, but alert.

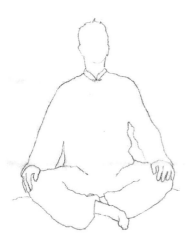

Figure 6. Sitting Meditation

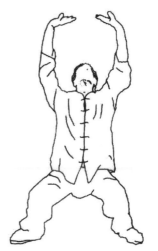

Figure 7. Standing Meditation

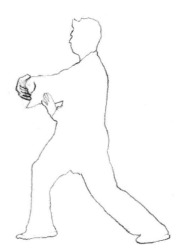

Figure 8. Moving slow meditation

time in this state, except during the few seconds right before we fall asleep. The untrained mind tends to stray toward activity and daydreaming, or deeper into the delta sleep state. Do not be discouraged, though, through knowledge and practice, this skill can be acquired.

Internal arts masters were aware of this problem for the beginning student. They developed postures and methods, tricks and secrets, to stay longer in the desired brainwave state. Sitting and chanting during meditation (Figure 6), standing and using visualizations such as in Yoga and *Qigong* (Figure 7), or moving slowly with a martial intention as in Tai Chi (Figure 8) are meant to help the student develop this ability or skill.

The reason that physical posture, mental technique, or even the sound of a bell is used is that through training with these methods, the student can practice attaining this state. Reaching this deep level of relaxation with a meditative mind sets up the correct environment for higher success in the martial arts, and is one of the key secrets of awakening the self-healing mechanisms within ourselves.

Physical Movements & Mental Visualizations

When teaching my students the movements, philosophy, and concepts of the various Eastern arts, and working with them on what I call "mind/body prescriptions" for healing or for martial arts, I often ask questions to sense their level of understanding. After years of teaching, I realized that my students usually gave me partial answers, addressing an issue either on a physical level or only the mental, but very rarely a complete answer. Therefore, I now ask them to give me a complete answer, or to answer by first acknowledging that the response is based on the physical or mental aspect. The reason why I am telling this story is to emphasize the importance of understanding both sides—the *Yang* physical body, and the *Yin* mental, or energetic, body. Both bodies are one and cannot be separated, but at some times they can be trained separately for better results.

Here is an example of a question that I hear from many students: What is happening when we are performing the Full and Empty Moon breathing? A good answer would be: On a physical level, we are moving the abdominal muscles and back muscles in and out as far as we can in a relaxed manner, coordinated with the movement of the perineum. Mentally, have a strong sensation of residing in the Center of Gravity Energy Center, and experience the three forces: Earth, Human, and Heaven.

Here we will take the time to explain the various internal visualization skills you will be utilizing during the preparation exercises and your Tai Chi practice. These visualizations are tools we will use increasingly throughout this book, and they are a fundamental aspect of your training which need be explored deeply before you move on to the Tai Chi form.

If you do not feel comfortable with more than two visualizations at the same time, your mind is not ready, and you have advanced through each stage of your training too quickly. The length of training of each stage is different for each individual. Take your time and enjoy each stage of developing these internal visualizations. Some days are better than others. Do not be too hard on yourself. Take each day of your training in stride. One day, you will find that your awareness of yourself, your surroundings, and the meaningfulness of your life have expanded greatly.

First Steps in the Journey of Internal Visualization

The first step that will help you to begin to become aware of both your physical and mental body is to sit cross-legged or on an edge of a chair (Figure 9) with proper alignment and experience the various basic energy centers, channels, and vessels that run through our bodies and distribute energy (*Qi*). Sitting this way allows you to focus on experiencing your torso. Once you are able to sense the movement of this *Qi* energy your sensations will become stronger, and you should move on to more advanced stages of internal visualizations with standing and moving postures, which include other energy concepts and work with channels in the limbs and the forces surrounding us.

Step 1: Physical Journey

Establish a good sitting foundation. The legs should be crossed comfortably if possible, or if the student is able to sit in a more advanced posture, you may sit in lotus position, with the right foot on the left thigh, and the left foot on the right thigh. You may also sit in half-lotus as your legs develop flexibility. Sit up straight on the edge of a cushion so gravity does not pull on your lower back and distract your mind. Though it can be difficult to re-train the muscles to sit up very straight and aligned, balancing the spine upon itself, slouching even slightly will cause a sore back very quickly. The edge of the knees should rest completely on the floor, to create a strong, triangular base, between the sitting bones in the rear and the outside of the knees. This posture will diminish the flow of energy in the legs, so you may begin to experience the

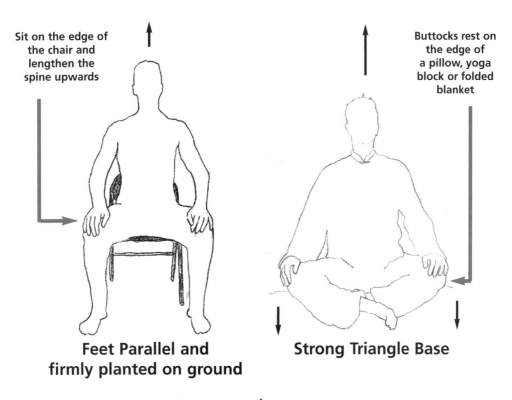

Sit on the edge of the chair and lengthen the spine upwards

Buttocks rest on the edge of a pillow, yoga block or folded blanket

Feet Parallel and firmly planted on ground

Strong Triangle Base

Figure 9. Two variations of correct sitting postures

energy in the torso, circulating in what is called the Microcosmic Orbit, or Small Circulation. Your energy naturally circulates down the front of your body from your navel, underneath, between the legs, and then up the center of the back and neck, over the top of the head, down the center of the face, and then down the front of the body to the navel again. Your tongue should touch the roof of your mouth, right behind the front teeth, to complete this circuit.

Step 2: Mental Journey

Follow the breath with your mind to calm the thoughts and reach a basic level of physical relaxation and awareness. Your complete attention should be continuously held on the breath as it moves in and out. This is the first requirement for training, as taught in Zen meditation, which is known as *Chan* in Chinese.

Physical & Mental Breath Work

When you inhale, feel your abdomen expanding to draw a breath, the breath entering the nose, moving the nose hairs, then moving to the back of the throat, to the bronchial tubes, and then filling the different sections of the lungs. Pay special attention to the feelings and sensations of the interactions between the air moving in and out and the body cells it is touching. Put your mind into each part of your body experiencing these sensations. Experience the end of inhalation and then linger for a moment before exhaling. This is considered the quietest time in our body. By training this skill of putting your mind into your body, you will develop a stronger and more sensitive mind/body connection, which will enable you to be aware of your health, and other aspects of your life, on a much more sensitive level.

During the exhale, feel how the air leaves the different areas of the lungs, out of the bronchial tubes, through the throat, past the nose hairs, and out the nose. Pay special attention to those feelings or sensations. Experience the end of inhalation. Linger again for a moment on this part of your breathing and try to sense other movement in your body while you are in this quiet, still place. This is called "looking for the motion in the stillness."

When you focus awareness (or Wisdom Mind, *Yi* in Chinese) entirely on the breath, you will help to create a state of No Thoughts. When random thoughts arise, simply observe them, with a neutral emotional state, and then turn your attention back to observing the breath. The Chinese call this state The Horse Mind Seizing the Monkey Mind. The breath should be long, quiet, peaceful, slender, continuous, and soft. Inhalation and exhalation should be balanced and equal in length, unless the student is in the more advanced stages of training in which we use the breath differently to change *Kan* (Water) and *Li* (Fire) in the body.

Step 3: Relaxing the physical body

The goal is to use only the minimum physical muscular force to hold and lengthen the spine in comfortable physical alignment. Let go of unnecessary tension in the entire body. One by one, relax your face, your shoulders, your arms, your torso, your belly, your hips, your legs, and your feet. Become aware of the up and down forces in the body during sitting meditation (Figure 10); the bones and muscles lifting and holding you up, while the shoulders and the soft tissue, including the face, are "melting" down as gravity pulls down on you. My teaching of this has been influenced by the teachings of students of Martha Graham and by the work described in various books, one of which is *Anatomy in Movement* by Blandine C. Germaine.

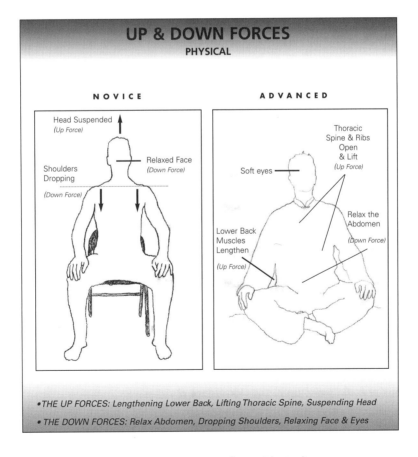

Figure 10. Up & Down forces (Physical)

Physical & Mental Combined

The torso of the body can be equated to three spheres resting on top of each other like a snowman (or snowwoman). Balancing these three spheres on top of a strong foundation is the first step toward experiencing physical transparency, which will help the mind "forget" the body and focus on reaching the required brainwave activity. Of course, in reality the body and mind cannot be separated.

Each sphere has an upward and downward force simultaneously occurring. The upward lifting feeling is usually associated with and encouraged during your inhale. The downward sinking/relaxing feeling is usually associated with and encouraged during your exhale. Once this pattern occurs naturally, you should try switching the combination of forces and breath to increase your internal control. When inhaling, emphasize the downward forces while monitoring and maintaining the upward forces, and when exhaling emphasize the up forces while monitoring and maintaining the downward forces.

THREE SPHERES

The three spheres correspond to the following body parts (Figures 11 and 12).

Sphere 1: The Lumbar Spine and Abdominal Muscles

The up force: Push into the sitting bones of the pelvis to allow the lumbar spine to open and start to lift upward. Do not push too much in the direction of the stomach. The downward force: Relax the abdominal muscles and the organs and start to feel a downward force. Concentrate on properly positioning this sphere before working on the next spheres. The legs should remain crossed, and may go numb, to slow down, but not stop, energy and blood circulation. Periodically uncross your legs and allow them to recuperate as your legs slowly become conditioned.

Sphere 2: The Thoracic Spine and Shoulders/Upper Back/Upper Chest

The up force: You want to lift up behind the sternum, the thoracic spine, to create a rising upward force. You also want to sink the chest slightly and arc the back into a "turtle back" so as not to have a militarily straight posture. The downward force: Relax the shoulders by pulling them horizontally outward and simultaneously downward at a 45-degree angle. Some individuals will also need to draw the shoulders gently backward. At first, check your alignment in a mirror until you can recognize the sensation of good posture.

Sphere 3: The Cervical Spine/Top of the Head/Face Muscles

The up force: You want to imagine a string gently pulling the top of the head, slightly lifting the cervical spine and skull. The downward force: You also want to relax and allow the muscles of the face to relax with a downward melting sensation.

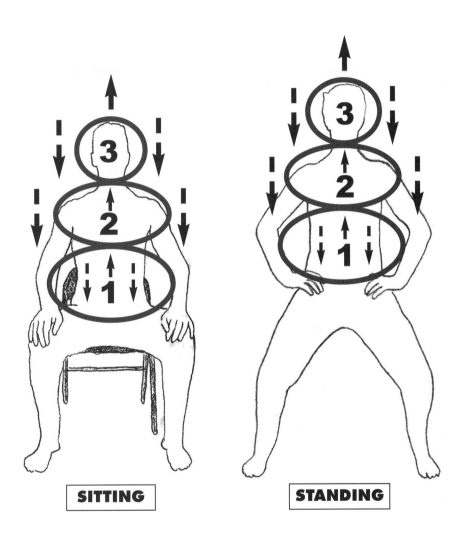

Figure 11. The Three Spheres (with the Up and Down forces)

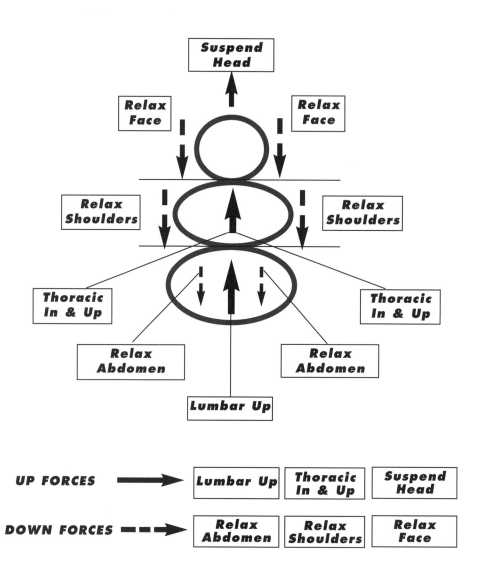

Figure 12. Three Spheres (with the Up and Down forces)

Please Note: There are also the minor up and down forces to become aware of in the body, such as the up force of gently lifting, or lengthening, through the spine, and the down force of relaxing the groin area. Another example of these minor forces is the up force of the air moving up the nostrils as we breathe in, while the down force of the relaxation of the nose, throat, and lungs takes place on a cellular level.

CENTER OF GRAVITY ENERGY CENTER

The main energy center of the body is located two inches below the belly button and about three inches inward from that same spot, in our physical Center of Gravity area. In *Qigong*, this area is known as the Lower *Dan Tian*, which translates as Elixir Field and is believed to be the main area of the body where *Qi* energy is stored and from where it is circulated. The first skill that is needed for both martial arts and health is the ability to reside mentally in the Center of Gravity Energy Center (Figure 13), while physically moving the abdomen and back muscles in and out with the breath. I refer to this controlled expansion and contraction of the abdomen and back muscles as Empty Moon and Full Moon (Figure 14). This is the secret to storing *Qi* energy, and upgrading our human battery in the center of our human electromagnetic field.

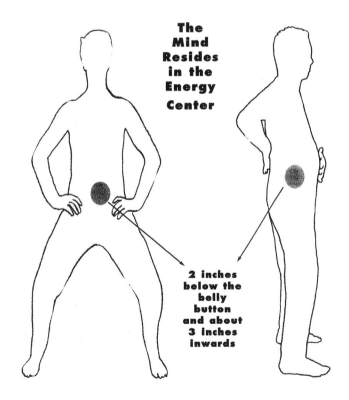

Figure 13. Center of Gravity Energy Center Breathing

The practice of residing in the Lower Energy Center should not only be an exercise. It should eventually be practiced throughout all your daily activities. There are many benefits that this skill will give you for martial and health training. In this section, we will focus on the training and not the theory. It is best not to fill the mind with too many concepts and thoughts, as we are trying to develop a more sensitive internal sense.

EMPTY & FULL MOON

Physically, we want to regain control over our abdominal and back muscles. Many of us have lost the firmness and control over those muscles. If you do not use it, you lose it. Starting to move them with the help of your hands, one on the back and one on the abdomen is the first step. The muscles can move in or out on either inhalation or exhalation. When they move out, it is Full Moon, and when they move inward, it is Empty Moon. At first, just breathe naturally and deeply, and move the muscles in and out with only 80 percent effort. You may initially experience little movement and control over the back and abdominal muscles, especially the back, which move significantly less. I compare the movement at this stage of training to the pulsing of the skin of a drum, just moving in and out without much control. As you progress, you will be able to move the muscles while counting 30 levels or stages between Full Moon and Empty Moon, meaning that you have developed excellent control over those muscles, and can imitate the actual cycle of the moon.

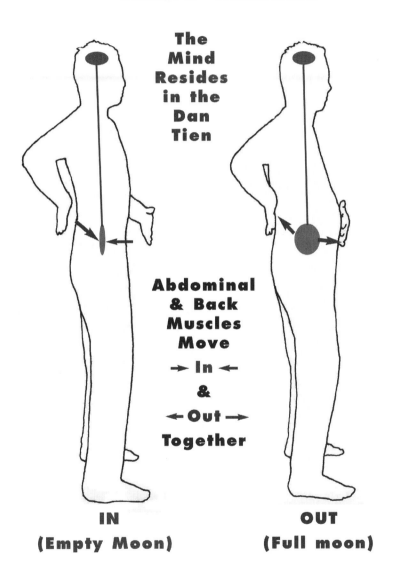

Figure 14. Center of Gravity Energy Center Breathing with Empty Moon/Full Moon

BUDDHIST BREATHING

On a physical level:

When inhaling, expand the abdominal and back muscles to Full Moon, and when exhaling, move the abdominal and back muscles in to Empty Moon.

On a mental level:

During this breathing, put your mind in the Lower Energy Center. The mind needs to reside there with the sensation of a point or a ball. At first when putting the mind in the center of gravity, your thoughts may pull your mind away, and you will find that you are thinking of something else entirely. The trick is not to fight this when it occurs, as it will often. The fact that the emotional Monkey Mind has stolen our Horse Mind away from being focused on our energy center is natural. Allow the mind to let the thoughts pass and return your awareness to the energy center. This kind of gentle looping visualization of the mind losing its focus and regaining it, without reacting emotionally (being disappointed that you lost your focus briefly) is an important trick.

Another trick is to place your hands on the abdomen and lower back (Figure 15), and visualize the spot between your two hands until you develop a strong sensation there. Yet another method of achieving this same focused awareness of mentally residing in the center of gravity is to drop an imaginary fishing line down the inside your body from the center of the top of your head, the Heavenly Gate, until it reaches the lower energy center. Each individual can find his or her own ways to reach the goal of mentally residing in our center of gravity energy center.

TAOIST BREATHING

On a physical level:

When inhaling, contract the abdominal and back muscles to Empty Moon, and when exhaling, expand the abdominal and back muscles out to Full Moon (Figure 15). Taoist breathing is more aggressive than Buddhist breathing and will help you to generate abundant *Qi* energy more quickly.

On a mental level:

Once you are able to reside in this center, start mentally pulsing the sensation of the ball of energy that you have created in your center of gravity. When inhaling, the ball shrinks, or condenses, and when exhaling the energy ball expands. Imagine that as it condenses and expands, it also glows brighter like a ball of light with a dimmer switch in your belly.

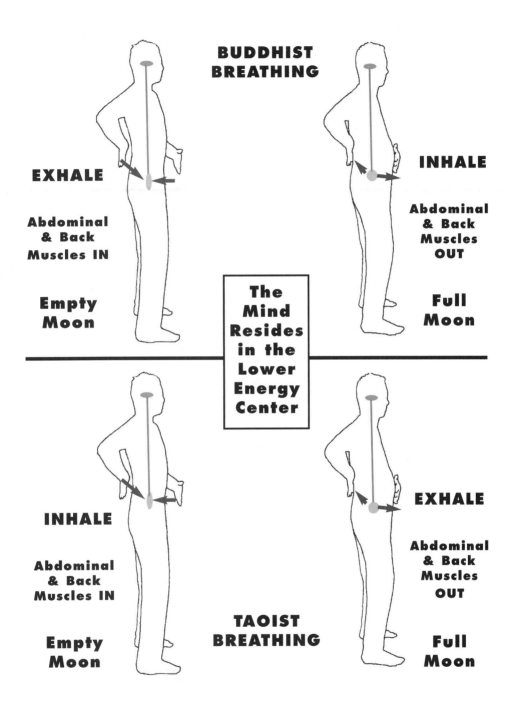

Figure 15. Buddhist and Taoist Breathing

There are two standing exercises which help bring the mind into the Center of Gravity Energy Center:

Exercise #1 is for two people: Stand with a Partner. Partner A places the center of one of his palms on the front of Partner B two inches below the belly button, and the other palm on Partner B's lower back muscles, near the kidneys (or Mingmen cavity in acupuncture).

As Partner A inhales, Partner B exhales, and vice versa. You exhale and your partner inhales. Both partners focus their attention on Partner B's center of gravity. At the same time, both partners imagine they are circulating energy through the Four Gates of the body, both palms and both feet.

Exercise #2: Stand with your knees slightly bent, legs shoulder-width apart. Place your palms, one on top of each other, two inches below the navel. Use Taoist breathing and imagine drawing energy up from the center of the molten core of the Earth. Lead the energy up into the two gates in the soles of the feet, up through the center of your legs, and into your Center of Gravity Energy Center. Exhale, allowing the mind and this energy to expand from the point in your energy center outward into the internal organs.

This is a mind/body prescription that I use with students and patients, which massages the internal organs from the outside, using the movements of the trunk muscles, and increases blood and oxygen circulation in the organs. I call this exercise Happy Organs.

PITUITARY GLAND ENERGY CENTER VISUALIZATION

The Pituitary Gland Energy Center is located under the two lobes of the brain in the center, in the middle of your head. See the diagram of the brain (Figure 16) to understand the exact location of the Pituitary Gland Energy Center; it is where the spinal cord connects to the base of the two brain lobes and the surrounding area, which includes the pituitary and pineal glands. Focus your entire mind into this area, as you did in the Lower Energy Center exercise, using the same visualization of a point or a ball of energy. Allow all your thoughts to dissipate, and focus only on this Upper Energy Center, as your breath moves slowly in and out.

Training the Pituitary Gland Energy Center is a little more difficult since it is closer to the brain cells. Leading energy into the brain is likely to activate more brain cells and cause more distraction for the Monkey Mind. However, there is a trick to help.

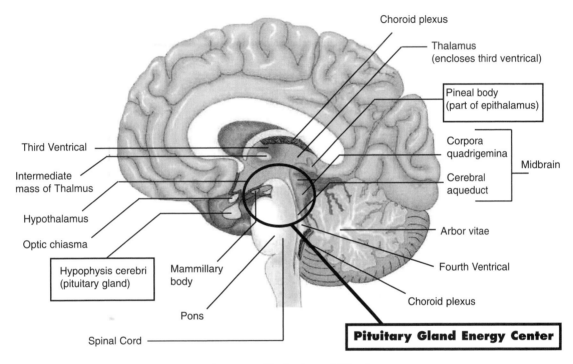

Choroid plexus

Thalamus
(encloses third ventrical)

Pineal body
(part of epithalamus)

Corpora
quadrigemina

Cerebral
aqueduct

Midbrain

Third Ventrical

Intermediate
mass of Thalmus

Hypothalamus

Optic chiasma

Hypophysis cerebri
(pituitary gland)

Mammillary
body

Arbor vitae

Fourth Ventrical

Choroid plexus

Pituitary Gland Energy Center

Pons

Spinal Cord

Figure 16. The Brain and Glands

EXTERNAL BATON VISUALIZATION

Hold one of your hands, or the Tai Chi ball (Figures 17 and 18), with a gently closed fist in front of your nose, directly in front of the Upper Energy Center location. Project the sensation of the fist or the ball inward to the pituitary gland area.

PROJECTING THE TAI CHI BALL
HELPS VISUALIZE ENERGY CENTERS

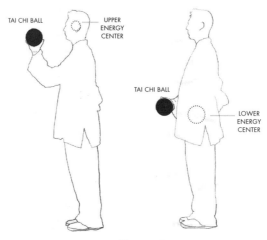

Figure 17.

PROJECTING THE TAI CHI BALL &
CREATING THE INTERNAL ENERGETIC BATON

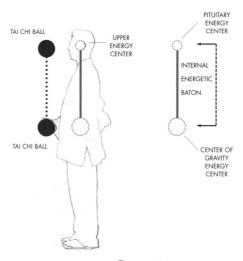

Figure 18.

BATON VISUALIZATION

Once you have been able to stay focused on both the upper and lower energy centers separately, you should then connect the two with a straight line through the center of the body, not the spine, like a baton (Figures 19 and 20). This sensation of a line through the center of the body will strengthen over time, as you develop a stronger sense of the relationship between the upper and lower energy centers. The pituitary gland energy center is the top head of the baton and the center of gravity energy center is the lower head of the baton. You can also use a more spiritual visualization like a baton made of light. One of the tasks I ask my students to tackle is to notice the various sensations of each of the energy centers, the balls of

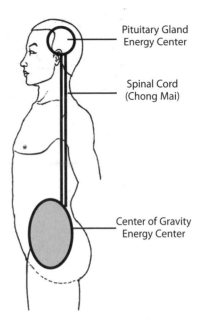

Figure 19. Diagram of Batons

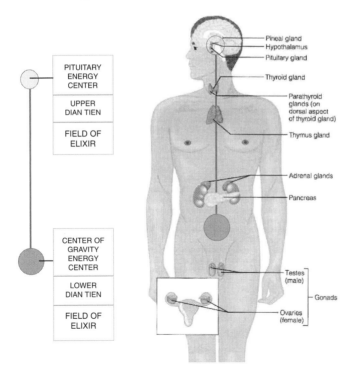

Figure 20. The Brain, the Glands, and the Baton

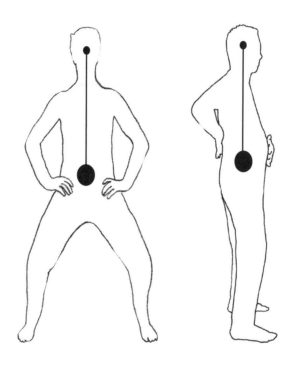

Figure 21. Baton Visualization

the baton, and to observe the similarities and differences in the sensations that are revealed during quiet observation of each one (see Figures 16, 18, 20, and 21).

Once you are able to maintain a strong visualization of the energy baton through the center of your body, try leading the energy from the top head of the baton down to the lower head of the baton energy center (Figure 22). As you progress, one day you may experience the sensation that you are sitting in the Lower Energy Center and looking up the baton toward the Upper Energy Center. You may sense the energy from the Upper Center dropping gently on top of you like rain falling. Some people experience a feeling like honey dripping down the outside and inside the body.

When you have an unusual experience during your practice, such as a sudden intensely pleasant sensation, try to let it pass without distracting you, and without "attaching" to it. If you practice while trying to have this experience or sensation again, it may hold you back and limit your progress.

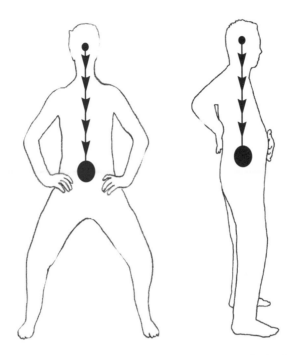

**Lead the energy from the upper ball of the baton
to the bottom ball.**

Figure 22. Baton Visualization—Quieting the Upper Energy Center

Bubble Visualization (Guardian Energy)

The bubble visualization is an easier one because it is outside our body. This skill can be acquired by visualizing a bubble around the physical body, about a fist away from the surface of the skin, like a cocoon (Figure 23). Some of my students sense they are within an egg, or they sense a fog or mist around them. Some experience this mist in many colors. Whatever visualization it takes to strengthen this sensation and awareness of a bubble surrounding the body is legitimate. In the beginning, you may experience holes or areas that are not as strong in the cocoon or the bubble as other areas. That is normal. Keep patching the weak parts of the bubble with your mind while maintaining and thickening the areas that are already strong. Over time you will have a thick and vibrant energy bubble around you that can be utilized for both martial and health goals. This energy is related to the Western concept of aura energy. In ancient times, the Chinese recognized this energy as *Wei Qi*, or Guardian Energy, and believed it to be an energetic component or reflection of our immune system.

BUBBLE VISUALIZATION

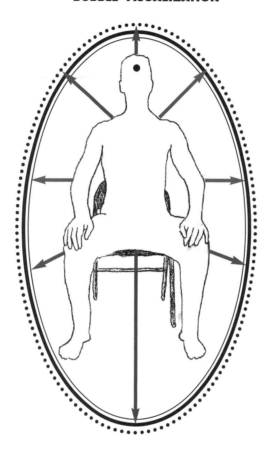

Figure 23.

BATON/BUBBLE BREATHING VISUALIZATION: (BONE MARROW-SKIN BREATHING)

Once you have created the baton and the bubble visualizations separately, start leading the mind from one visualization to the other, or from one place to the other. When inhaling, bring the energy of your entire body inward with your mind from the bubble to the baton in the center of your body. When exhaling, use your mind to lead energy from the baton back outwards into the bubble (Figure 24). You can do this with either breathing technique, Taoist or Buddhist. Once you have a strong ability to maintain the baton/bubble visualization, try to develop the skill further and

BATON•BUBBLE BREATHING VISUALIZATION

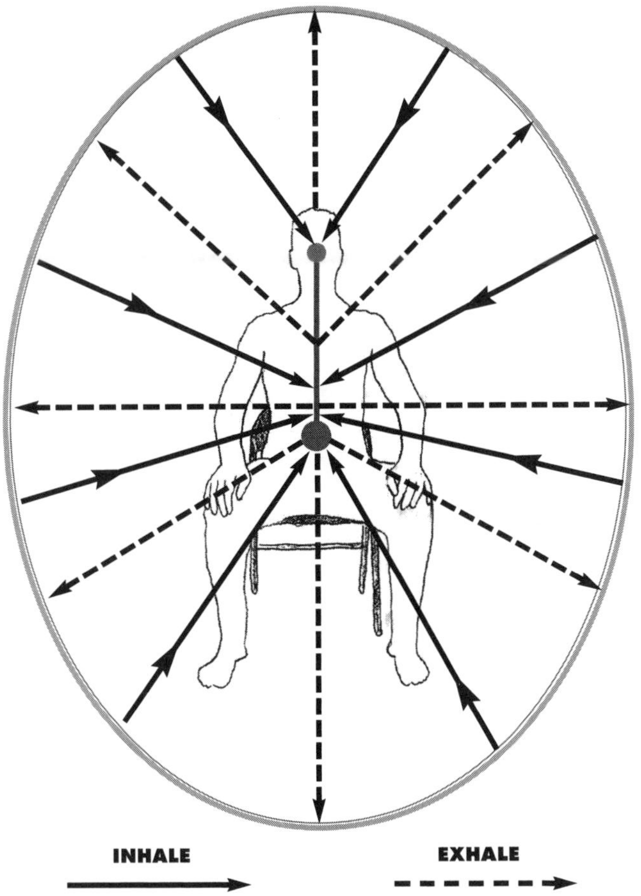

INHALE   **EXHALE**

Figure 24 Baton/Bubble Breathing

be aware of the bubble as you inhale to the baton, and vice versa. The two are one, but still are two. In reality, they cannot be separated.

A caution with this exercise: if you practice drawing your energy inward towards the baton, and you shrink your Guardian Energy during a time when you are exposed to negative elements such as cold winter air, you may lower your immune system and get sick more easily. To avoid this, practice until you can sense that when you draw your energy inward, you still maintain the strong bubble visualization surrounding your body.

FOUR GATES BREATHING

We have five major energy gates in our body and many other small ones. In fact, each of your skin's pores can be considered a gate on a small scale. The five gates are the head, the center of the palms, and the soles of the feet. In our training, we will work with the hands and feet (Figure 25). I recommend that in the beginning, and occasionally at other times, you train only two gates at a time. When inhaling, the ball of energy at the center of our Gravity Energy Center squeezes into a focused ball, but at the same time the energy from that ball rises up in the back through the Governing Vessel. The Governing Vessel is an energy path on the back of the torso

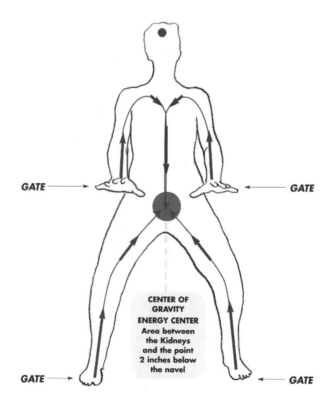

GATE

GATE

GATE

GATE

CENTER OF GRAVITY ENERGY CENTER
Area between the Kidneys and the point 2 inches below the navel

LEAD THE MIND FROM THE 4 GATES
TO THE CENTER OF GRAVITY ENERGY CENTER

Figure 25. Four Gates Breathing (Inhalation)

that runs upwards between the spine and the skin on our back. The mind leads the energy upward to the area between the shoulder blades while inhaling, and then during the exhalation, the mind leads the energy out from the shoulder blade area, out through the arms, and through the fingers and the center of the palms. At the same time, the mind leads the energy from the focused energy ball in the Center of Gravity down through the legs, and out through the toes and the soles of our feet.

You may notice that the visualizations through the lower gates are simpler. The mind just focuses on leading the energy from the energy ball at the Lower Energy Center down and out of the feet during the exhale, and back up again during the inhale. The visualization through the upper gates is more complex and that is why I recommend first practicing two gates at a time. The mind needs to use one inhale to reach the shoulder blades area and the following exhale to lead the energy out through the palms and fingers.

Once you feel comfortable with this path of visualization, add the last piece of the Four Gates breathing. When inhaling, also lead energy inward through the palms up through the inner arm and down the front of the body back to the lower energy center. Your mind is required to visualize more then one visualization simultaneously. I call this multi-visualizing. You will practice this until it becomes a natural, effortless sensation. As you lead energy through these pathways of the body, the pathways will gradually widen, and your ability to have a stronger sensation of what is happening in these channels, meridians, and vessels will become much more sensitive.

This is the stage of Regulating without Regulating, or fine-tuning until fine-tuning is not needed, at which time you can again simply focus your awareness on maintaining a neutral state of mind, and mentally reach the place of the Thought of No Thought. Four Gates breathing is the basic breathing technique that should be used throughout all of your Tai Chi practice. As you can see, this can take a long time to develop to a high level of proficiency.

THIRD EYE/SPIRITUAL BREATHING

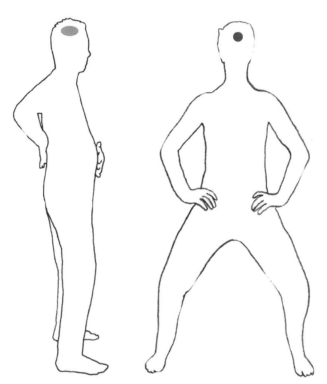

**The third eye is right behind the middle of the
forehead, in front of the two brain lobes.**

Figure 26. The Spiritual Valley

THIRD EYE PULSING OR SPIRITUAL BREATHING

Spiritual breathing, at first, is simply residing with the mind in the Third Eye area
in the center of your forehead. It is right behind the front of the skull, in front of the
space between the two lobes of the brain. This space is known as the Spiritual Valley
in *Qigong* (Figure 26). The mind resides in a fixed point in this Third Eye area while
"cooling" down the energy of the eyes and brain. When you cool the energy of the eyes
and brain, the third eye or spiritual breathing is stronger and clearer (Figure 27). This
gate is also the path we lead the Sun into to nourish our entire being and to boost our

THIRD EYE/SPIRITUAL BREATHING

Cooling Down the Excess Eye & Brain Energy

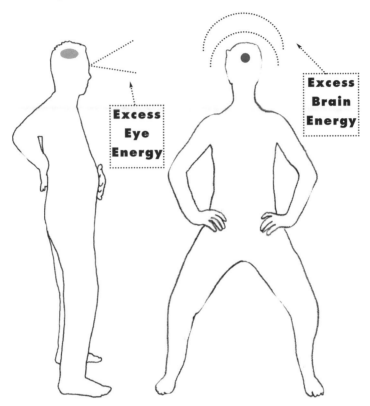

Excess Eye Energy

Excess Brain Energy

The third eye is right behind the middle of the forehead, in front of the two brain lobes.

Figure 27 Third Eye/Spiritual Breathing (Cooling down the excess eye and brain energy)

energetic system (Figure 28). You may have a sensation of pressure in this area. As one of my teachers told me, do not be too quick to attempt to reopen the Third Eye. This may occur naturally only after many years of diligent training, of both the physical body, and of the neutral and peaceful state of mind. People in the West are quick to speak of opening the Third Eye or of attaining enlightenment, but in fact, these experiences are not only metaphysical events—they are physiological processes which take many years to develop, and are quite difficult, even for a mighty sage of ancient times.

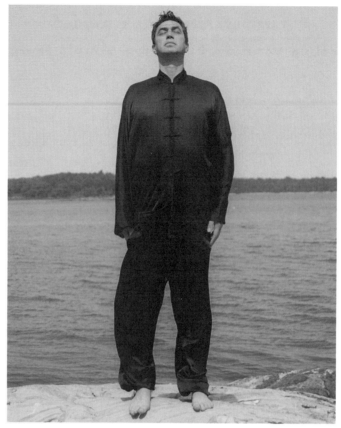

Figure 28. Tapping into abundant sun energy, boosting our energetic system

BATON/BUBBLE AND FOUR GATES SPIRITUAL BREATHING

When you feel comfortable with each visualization separately, you may then practice them combined as a whole. This can only be done once they have been trained, regulated, and fine tuned to a degree where constant monitoring is no longer necessary. When combining, you may find it mentally difficult to have complete visualization happening at the same time. Expect to act more like the conductor of an orchestra; your mind is aware of all visualizations, but it moves naturally between them, while staying a deeply relaxed state.

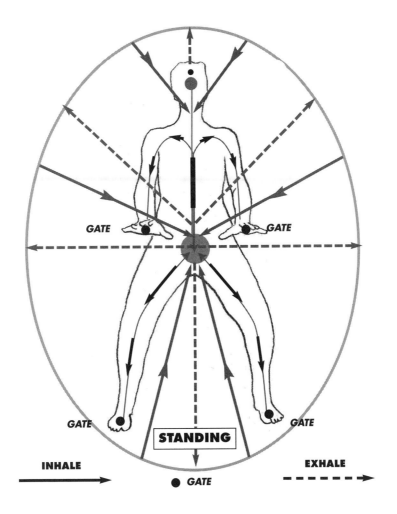

Figure 29. Four Gates with Baton/Bubble Breathing Visualization—Standing

Inhale and focus on leading the mind inward from the bubble to the baton, while noticing the energy that is condensed at the Lower Energy Center and its movements up the spine. Focus, while sitting or standing, for a minute or two on the Empty Moon and Full Moon, while remaining aware, in the back of your mind, of the Four Gates, your energetic baton, as well as your energetic bubble (Figures 29 and 30).

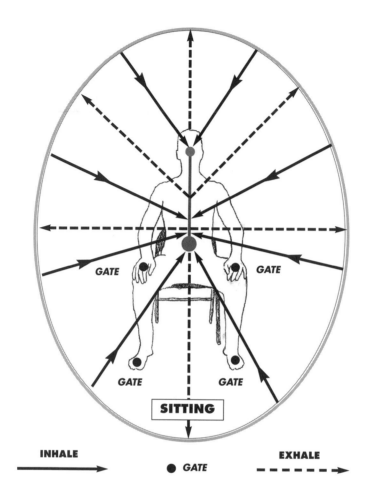

Figure 29. Four Gates with Baton/Bubble Breathing Visualization—Sitting

Some days when I sit or stand, this is how I train the various visualizations: During a 45-minute session, I set a chime for five minutes, and then I train my awareness of the up and down forces for five minutes while also "surfing" the breath; I spend five minutes emphasizing Empty and Full Moon; five minutes residing in the Lower Center of Gravity Energy Center; five minutes residing in the Pituitary Gland Upper Energy Center; five minutes strengthening the baton; five minutes building the bubble; five minutes of baton/bubble breathing, and then the rest of the time, or during other sittings, I monitor, or conduct, peacefully moving my focus quietly from one to the other, yet keeping my awareness on them as a whole.

CHAPTER 3
Sunrise Tai Chi Mind/Body Program

Now we will work on some preparation exercises to stretch and warm up the physical body for our practice of Tai Chi. In my experience, it is best to build up to the point where one can hold each stretch for three minutes to allow the cells in the tissue you are working with reach an excited state. After three minutes, the cells of the muscles and tendons are "ready" to allow real change to take place.

It is recommended to move and shift position slowly. Remember, if you are breathing, you are moving. Try to become aware of the difference between constructive pain and destructive pain. These sensations are your body's way of communicating its needs to your mind. Respect these sensations, and allow the tissues the time needed to stretch very gradually. Use your mind to monitor the different muscles you are working with; notice which muscles tense and which ones relax, and over time this skill will improve.

Remember: Each of the exercises is comprised of physical skills and mental visualizations. Practice each one separately, and once you are comfortable with each, combine them.

1. SITTING MEDITATION

Breathe deeply. Look for the motion in the stillness. Practice your internal visualization at whatever stage of the training to which you have progressed. While facing the direction of the sunrise, relax your entire body, keeping your spine straight, and your head suspended.

Remember: This meditation does not have to be done outdoors or exactly at sunrise.

The energy from the sun and our surroundings can be absorbed through walls and windows. Of course, the soft light before and during sunrise as the natural *Yin* becomes *Yang* will offer the optimal experience.

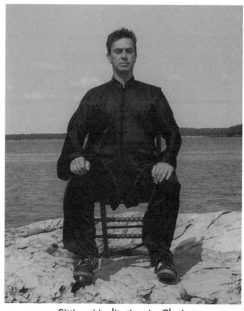

Sitting Meditation in Chair

Be aware that as we age, we become shallow breathers. We want the abdomen to move, as we breathe deeply, gently, and quietly. If you slouch and collapse your spine, you may utilize only a third of your lung capacity. When you keep your spine straight and long, you create space for the internal organs, and you allow more air to move in and more oxygen to nourish the entire body. In addition, you reduce stress on the vertebrae, and create space for the organs, making the organs happy, versus compressed and stagnant. I would recommend that you sit on the floor as described earlier, or on a firm chair or bed. A firm seated position will give you the foundation needed for lengthening the body, from the sitting bones up. I like to refer to this posture as the Emperor/Empress position (illustrated in the Sun Nourishing section), which symbolizes a strong, yet calm, spirit.

Relax your entire body and allow the warmth of the sun to absorb into the Third Eye area. Lead the energy inward to your Upper Energy Center in the middle of your brain. As you breathe deeply, allow the energy to expand outward, nourishing the entire brain.

Once you have a strong sensation of your Upper Energy Center, drop an imaginary line down through the middle of your body to your Lower Energy Center, an inch or two below your navel, into your physical Center of Gravity Energy Center.

Relax the entire face. You want to allow all of the soft tissue on your face and head to "melt" from the top down. Imagine the temple area melting down. You want to first relax the areas that are closer to the face bones. Relax the corners of the mouth and the corners of your nose. Melt and dissolve your cheeks and the corners of your eyes. After you finish dissolving and melting the tight areas in the face, imagine all the skin melting down, layer by layer, like an onion. Imagine you have ten layers in your face, and you allow each layer to dissolve. Often, we hold tension in our face that we are not aware of, which can cause headaches, TMJ (temporomandibular joint arthritis),* or high blood pressure.

START WITH 3 MINUTES, AND INCREASE YOUR TRAINING TIME GRADUALLY.

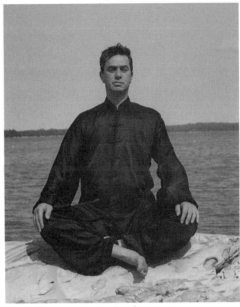

Sitting Meditation
(Advanced Posture)

---

*Temporomandibular joint arthritis: The temporomandibular joints are complex and are composed of muscles, tendons, and bones. When the muscles are relaxed and balanced and both jaw joints open and close comfortably, we are able to talk, chew, or yawn without pain. It is one of the most frequently used of all the joints in the body.

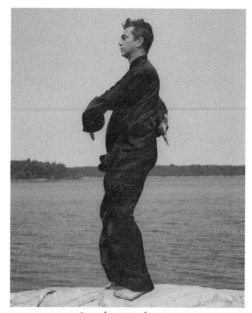

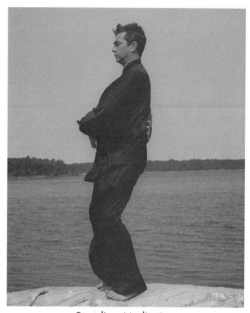

Standing Meditation
(Center of Gravity Energy Center Breathing)

Standing Meditation
(Center of Gravity Energy Center Breathing)

2. STANDING MEDITATION

Center of Gravity Breathing

Relax and experience a strong sensation of your Lower Energy Center. As you breathe deeply, allow the abdomen to move in and out, using either the Buddhist or Taoist breathing taught in the earlier section on internal visualizations. You may think of your expanded belly as a Full Moon, and when it is drawn in, it is an Empty Moon. Over the years, most of us use the abdominal muscles less and we lose control over them. Using the palm physically to reinforce the movement will help until the muscles can move independently. Eventually, when you can control those muscles without your hands, you will find out that they can even move in a wave, as opposed to the skin of drum that just moves in and out.

As a beginner, you will just move the muscles in and out. As you become more advanced, and have more control over the abdominal and lower back muscles, they will move in a wave. The wave starts from the bottom and goes up towards the solar plexus, and then it moves back downward. In the future, as your sensitivity develops, it will be easier to sense the wave motion within the back muscles on a smaller scale.

Your challenge is to try to count about thirty stages between Empty Moon and Full Moon, just like a lunar phase chart. It may take a while training this technique

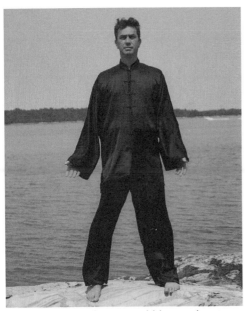

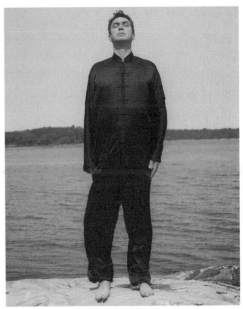

Standing Meditation (Bubble Breathing) Standing Meditation (Bubble Breathing)

to be able to do so within one breath. Doing so will show that you have control over those muscles. In addition, by moving these muscles you are massaging your organs. You are leading oxygen-rich blood and energy into them, and you are moving impurities and blood away from them.

START WITH 3 MINUTES, AND INCREASE YOUR TRAINING TIME GRADUALLY. PRACTICE EACH ENERGY CENTER VISUALIZATION SEPARATELY, UNTIL YOU CAN PUT THEM TOGETHER COMFORTABLY.

Bubble Breathing

During bubble breathing, condense the energy in your energy centers as you inhale. When you exhale, expand the energy outward, filling the entire body to the surface of the skin, and beyond. In this standing meditation, you want to experience a heavy sensation from your Center of Gravity down into your root, with a grounded feeling, while experiencing an opposite force, or a light feeling, moving up through the spine. This emphasis allows the Guardian Energy to expand wider naturally, and to be stronger for both health and martial arts.

Inhale, and draw your energy inward, returning it to your center. Then, exhale expanding outward from the center to form a bubble mentally around your body.

START WITH 3 MINUTES, AND INCREASE YOUR TRAINING TIME GRADUALLY.

3. CLEANSING THE BODY

As you inhale, raise your arms and slowly scan the inside of your body with your mind, from the feet up to the head. Bring the mind through the entire body, plateau by plateau and collect any impurities. Exhale and lead the impurities up and out through the palms.

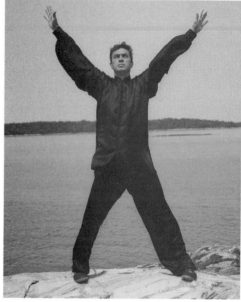

Deposit the impurities in the stars, far away. When we talk about impurities, we mean aches, pains, or anything that attracts your attention. Numbness, tingling, an uncomfortable feeling, or something you know is there.

Remember, you still want to maintain the sensation, or the imagery, of the energy centers. Keep your mind in the area of the pituitary and pineal glands, and in the center of gravity, also.

The mind slowly scans inside the entire physical body, collecting those impurities, and depositing them in the stars. The idea is that a lot of the stress and traumas that we go through in our lives are stored on a physical level somewhere

Cleansing the Body

in the soft tissue and the organs. We want to dissolve those impurities, or dissolve those traumas, or areas that stagnate energy, and lead them out of the body.

Maintain deep breath throughout the exercise. Relax your face, and your shoulders. Distribute the weight between the ball of the foot and the heels. Slightly bend your knees, which will also build up strength in your legs. Tuck the tailbone in slightly and maintain a peaceful, quiet, happy mind.

START WITH 3 MINUTES, AND INCREASE YOUR TRAINING TIME GRADUALLY.

4. NOURISHING THE BODY

Inhale and draw in clean, healthy energy from your surroundings. Allow the energy to pour into your body through the top of the head and to fill the body, plateau by plateau. Nourishing is similar in practice to cleansing, except we are now drawing energy into the body from our surroundings.

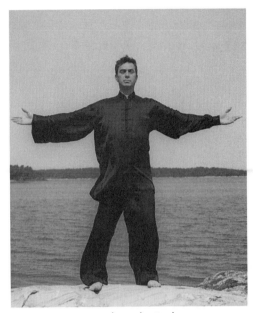

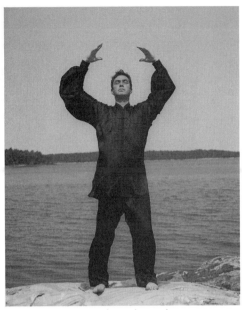

Nourishing the Body

Nourishing the Body

Slightly bend your knees. Tuck the tailbone in. Head suspended. Drop your shoulders. Breathe deeply so you can sense the ribs expanding. Connect mentally to the baton.

Sense the relationship of your body to the earth. Sense the relationship of your body to the heavens. Then, connect with your mind, through your fingers, to the earth. Draw the earth energy into your fingers. Draw the tree energy into your fingers. Draw in the mountain energy. Draw in the ocean energy. Draw in the sky energy, and draw in the energy of the stars and the heavens.

Lead all this energy into the body and funnel it down through the Heavenly Gate, which is the softer part on the very top of the head. Slowly lead the energy and sense how it is pouring into you, filling you up plateau by plateau.

Breathe deeply through the nose. Again, connect to the earth, connect to the trees, connect to the mountains and oceans, connect to the sky and the heavens, the stars, and lead all that energy, funnel it down, through the top of the head, the Heavenly Gate, to nourish the entire body, plateau by plateau.

Again, try to experience the heavy force from the Lower Energy Center down, and the light force, from the Center of Gravity up through the spine. One day you will be able to differentiate between the two more clearly. You will find out that

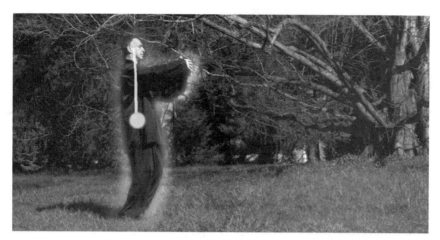

Embrace the Tree with Baton Visualization

when you inhale, you encourages the light force through the spine, and when you exhale, you encourages the heavy force through the legs. As you progress, you can emphasize the heavy force through the legs during exhalation, and when you inhale, emphasize the light force through the spine.

When nourishing, the experience of connecting to the forces of nature is very important. You may need to remember experiences or sensations that you have had with each one of those forces. For example, when you draw from the earth energy, perhaps you have had the experience of working in the garden, digging into the earth with your hands, feeling the soil, planting, seeing the results of planting, the growth.

For the tree energy, in the Eastern arts we have an exercise called Embrace the Tree, in which you metaphorically or literally hug a tree in order to exchange energy with it. Remember times you have walked or hiked through the forest, when you have hiked through the mountains. Sense that connection to the mountains. Perhaps you have stood at the top of a mountain, looking out over the land or sea.

All these experiences will allow you to experience a stronger sensation of each one of the forces which you draw energy from during this exercise. Connect not just with your imagination, but also with your emotions, and with your spirit. In doing so, the results and the benefits are much stronger, which in turn leads to better health and a higher quality of life.

The second aspect of this exercise is the sensation, or feeling, that you experience through the inside of the body, and outside on the skin, when you nourish the body. You may sense, or feel, as if you are taking a shower; a tingling sensation like water, internally as well as externally. This means you are achieving the goals that I am challenging you to reach. I am looking for you to develop the ability to scan the entire body, inside and out.

You will also develop the ability of being able to "connect" to the skin, to the fasciae, to the tendons and ligaments, to the bones, and most importantly, to the internal organs, allowing you to nourish the spine and the brain. It will take time and diligent practice to achieve this the ability of leading the mind to the desired area in the body and residing in it, eventually bringing you to the level at which you consciously stimulate healing action to take place.

START WITH 3 MINUTES, AND INCREASE YOUR TRAINING TIME GRADUALLY.

5. ORGAN MASSAGE

We massage our organs in two ways. One way of massaging the organs is through movements. The other way is literally through self-massage using your hands. This can be done standing or sitting.

Sit up straight and relax. Rub your hands until warm. While breathing deeply, massage the internal organs from right to left in a circular, spiraling motion. Repeat this circular motion three times. Then rub your hands again, and repeat the massage.

This massage should always follow the clockwise direction of the intestines. You want to help encourage that movement. If reversed, it can cause constipation, and is not recommended. Calm your mind and reach deep into the sensation of the baton.

Next, you want to monitor the up and down forces. Is your spine nice and straight? Are your shoulders relaxed? Is the top of the head suspended, and did you relax the entire face?

Put your mind inside the organs. You want to have the sense of smiling organs, happy organs. You want to have a sensation of nourishing the organs. You want to feel the sensation of relaxation in the organs, and of feeding them with good, healthy, pure energy.

START BY MASSAGING THE ORGANS FOR 3 MINUTES, AND INCREASE YOUR TIME GRADUALLY.

6. THREE CHAMBERS BREATHING

The lungs do not have muscle tissue that can be consciously controlled. They are like a balloon, and they must be compressed and expanded by the motion of the diaphragm and the muscles inside and outside the ribs. To gain control of these muscles, imagine that the lungs are made of three quadrants, or chambers, from bottom to top. The bottom layer is the first chamber. The middle of the lungs is the second, and the top of the lungs is the third.

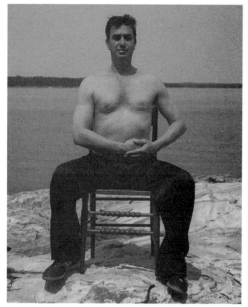

Organ Massage (Sitting)

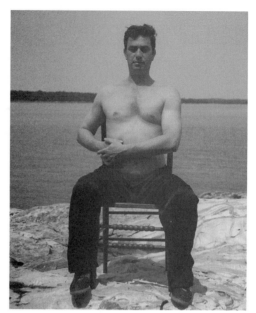

Organ Massage (Sitting)

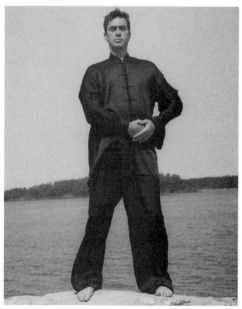

Organ Massage (Standing)

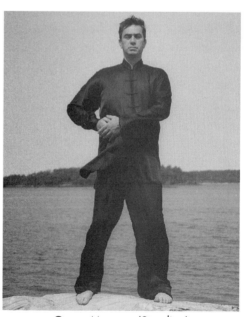

Organ Massage (Standing)

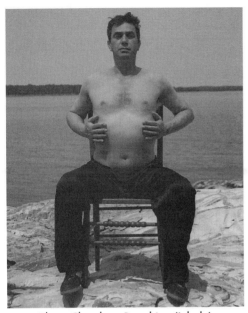
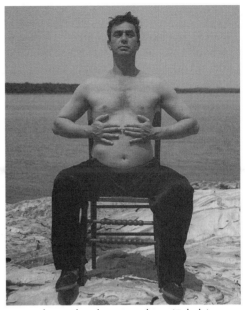

Three Chambers Breathing (Inhale)   Three Chambers Breathing (Exhale)

First, try to lead air into the bottom part of your lungs, which are near ribs eleven and twelve, the floating ribs. When you do this correctly, you will see and feel the floating ribs move sideways.

Then, fill chamber two, which is right beneath the chest.

Lastly, fill chamber three, the chest area.

When exhaling, empty the chambers one by one.

Visualize that you are breathing into these separate chambers in the front part of your lungs. You may choose to start by working with just one or two chambers, and once you are comfortable you may work with all three.

Our goal is to increase the lung capacity to take in more oxygen, which is vital for all of the body's functions on a cellular level.

START WITH 3 MINUTES, AND INCREASE YOUR TRAINING TIME GRADUALLY.

7. VITAMIN L – LOWER BACK STRETCH

This movement, like the others, can be practiced at a basic, intermediate, or more advanced level, either on the edge of a seat or on the floor, depending upon your level of flexibility. Once you have achieved the basic movements and stretches, you may then move on to a more challenging level.

Stretching the lower back and stimulating the kidney is one of the most important exercises one can do for health, and for martial arts training. I call this exercise Vitamin L because everybody takes their vitamins religiously, but they sometimes neglect this important exercise. Therefore, it has this nickname to motivate students to do it more consistently, on a daily basis.

For the first, or basic, level of this exercise, sit on the edge of a chair. Drop your head, and support your forehead on some surface, such as the edge of a bed. You want to be able to breathe comfortably through your nose. Lengthen the spine, so that you have a straight sensation through the spine, rather than a curved sensation.

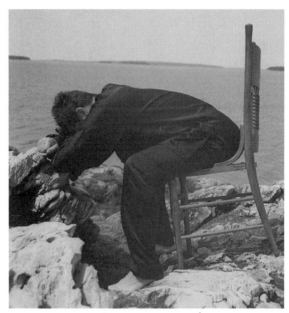

Vitamin L – Lower Back
(Straight forward: Beginner)

When you stretch the lower back, the muscles tense around the kidney area. When you release the stretch, the muscles release around the kidney area. Blood and energy circulation are slowed when the muscles are tensed and when the muscles relax, they are released, causing a gentle internal massage.

After sixty seconds of stretching the lower back straight forward (twelve o'clock), stretch the left side (ten o'clock) for sixty seconds, and then change and stretch the other side (two o'clock) for sixty seconds.

The second level of this exercise is for people who are more flexible,

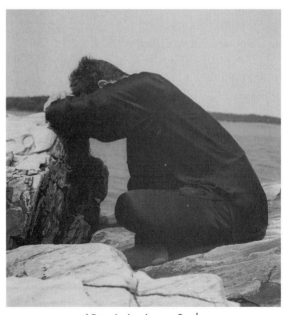

Vitamin L – Lower Back
(Straight forward: Advanced)

or for whom this stretch is no longer a challenge. Do the exercise as above, but sit on the floor, on a cushion or mat. Again, rest your head on something elevated off the floor at a comfortable height. This stretch also increases leg and groin flexibility, as well as the outer hip.

You may use your fists, your palms, or your arms to achieve this height as well. In addition, putting the arms forward adds to the force of the stretch. Remember, you always want to stretch at 80 percent of your capability, which is the key to avoiding injuries and advancing forward as fast and as safe as possible.

The advanced level of this exercise is, again, the same, except it is done on the floor with the elevation of the head

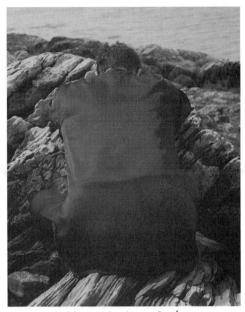

Vitamin L – Lower Back
(Straight forward or 12:00)

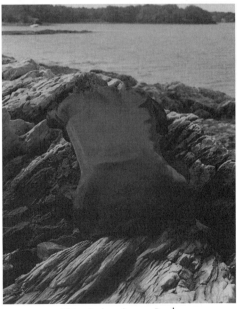

Vitamin L – Lower Back
(left side or 10:00)

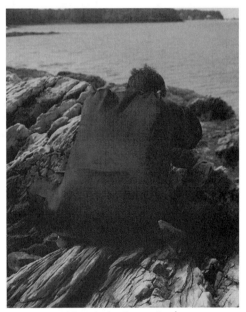

Vitamin L – Lower Back
(right side or 2:00)

removed. Simply rest your head and arms on the floor in front of you. Be careful in working up to this level of flexibility.

START WITH 3 MINUTES, AND INCREASE YOUR TRAINING TIME GRADUALLY, WHILE BEING CAREFUL NOT TO OVERDO IT.

8. FOUR GATES BREATHING

Stand and practice your Four Gates breathing as we discussed in the section on internal visualizations. Inhale, condense the Upper and Lower Energy Centers, and at the same time, lead the energy from your Lower Energy Center up along the spine in the Governing Vessel to the area between the shoulder blades.

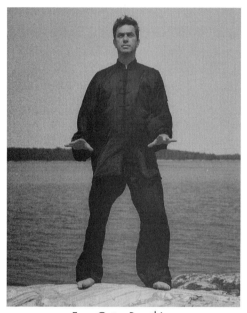

Exhale, lead the energy down through the arms and legs, and out through the Four Gates in the center of your palms and the soles of your feet.

Over time, you will develop this skill so that when you inhale, you will also draw energy in through the Four Gates, up the limbs, and into the baton in your energy center.

This training builds total body aware-ness, which has many physical benefits. At first, there is a tendency to have a stronger sensation in the upper two Gates (in the palms), but eventually you will be able to balance sensation evenly throughout all

Four Gates Breathing

Four Gates. Remember to lead the energy, rather than "pushing" it. Eventually, while the mind is in your Four Gates, it still senses your center, and when your mind is in your center, it still senses the Four Gates.

START WITH 3 MINUTES, AND INCREASE YOUR TRAINING TIME GRADUALLY.

9. TWO BOWS BREATHING

In this breathing exercise, we emphasize the stretching and releasing of the two major bows (out of the six) in our body: The chest, the crossbow, and the spine, the longbow.

Inhale and stretch the bows, slightly arching the upper back, tucking in the tailbone, and drawing in the chest. Exhale and release the bows. You may also stretch the bows in the opposite direction.

Once you feel confident that you can isolate the physical aspect of stretching the two bows, then add the visualizations of Four Gates breathing and Bubble breathing. START WITH 3 MINUTES; ONE AND A HALF MINUTES FOR EACH BOW, AND INCREASE YOUR TRAINING TIME GRADUALLY.

10. TAI CHI BALL

On a physical level, the Tai Chi Ball is used as a tool to strengthen the body.* As the arms lift this weight in front of the body, the lower back is exercised. This movement teaches coordination, fluidity, and the connection of the entire body from the soles of the feet to the tips of the fingers as a single, whip-like unit.

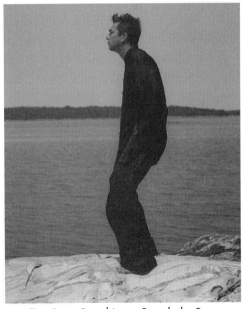

Two Bows Breathing – Stretch the Bow

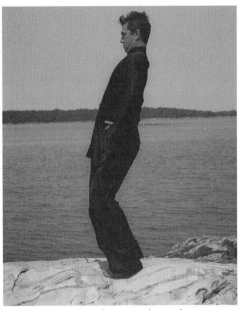

Two Bows Breathing – Release the Bow

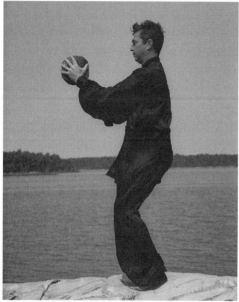

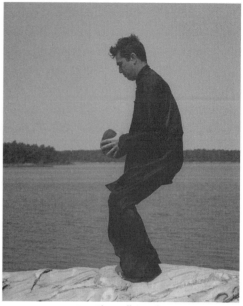

Tai Chi Ball (Rock)   Tai Chi Ball (Rock)

Mentally, the ball is a tool for the mind to strengthen the visualization of the balls of the baton, or the upper and lower energy centers. Through projecting the sensation of the ball internally, one can have a stronger visualization in a shorter time.

This is again an opportunity to practice the earlier skills of stretching and releasing the bows, and visualizing the Four Gates breathing. The movement of the external Tai Chi Ball corresponds to the internal energetic circulation in the body, and it will allow you to strengthen your sensation of the Upper and Lower Energy Centers. Notice the change in sensation in the energy centers as the Tai Chi Ball passes near them.

In traditional Tai Chi Ball training, the practitioner eventually develops the skill of passing *Qi* energy through the ball with the hands.

You may sit or stand. Circle the ball vertically for one and a half minutes forward and again for one and a half minutes backwards. Some days, you may also try rotating the ball horizontally clockwise, and then counterclockwise.

START WITH 3 MINUTES, AND INCREASE YOUR TRAINING TIME GRADUALLY.

11. VITAMIN H – HAMSTRING STRETCH

Tilt the pelvis upward. Breathe deeply, with long, calm, quiet, peaceful inhalation. Bend at the waist, until you feel an even stretch through your hamstrings and calf muscles. The leg muscles should be active or engaged; do not lock or hyperex-

---

*The preferred balls are usually made of wood which helps transmit the Qi energy through the ball between the hands. Other types of balls may be used such as bowling balls or soccer balls. First start with lighter balls, and then progress to heavier balls.

tend the knees. The spine is relaxed. Some times, you can shift your weight to the ball of the foot to stretch the calf muscles further. Raise your kneecaps slightly using your thigh muscles (quadriceps) to protect your knees.

The hamstrings are the most stubborn muscle in the body because they are used all day to support the weight of the entire body. When stretching, remember to use your mind to delve deeper and deeper into the layers of soft tissue in your body. This skill will improve over time.

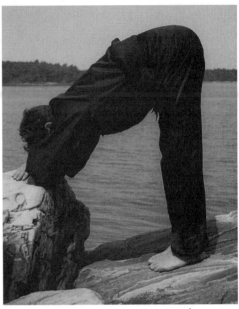
Vitamin H – Hamstring Stretch

Again, this exercise can be trained in three stages. First, start with resting your head on some surface for support. Then, gradually lower the supporting surface. Eventually, you will be bending and reaching the floor. If this advanced level of reaching the floor does not provide much of a stretch for you because the hamstrings are conditioned, try generating leverage by grabbing the back of your ankles, and pulling gently, or even by cupping your heels with your palms.

START WITH 3 MINUTES, AND INCREASE YOUR TRAINING TIME GRADUALLY, WHILE BEING CAREFUL NOT TO OVERDO IT.

12. LOOSENING LEG JOINTS

Loosen the hips, knees, and ankles. Circle each leg, one at a time, by pivoting on the toe. Circle outward, and then change the direction and circle inward. You can focus the movement into the ankle, or increase the range of movement to include the knee and hip.

Eventually you may also add the visualizations of Cleansing and Nourishing the entire body by leading energy through the legs. When the leg rotates outwards, pivoting on the toe, use the mind to scan the plateaus in the body and deposit any impurities into the earth.

When the legs rotate inward, draw energy up the leg from the earth using your Center of Gravity breathing, and release the accumulated pure energy into your internal organs.

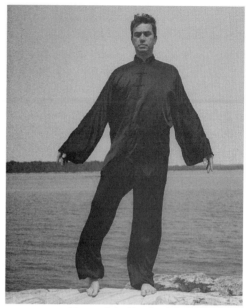

Hip and Ankles (right)

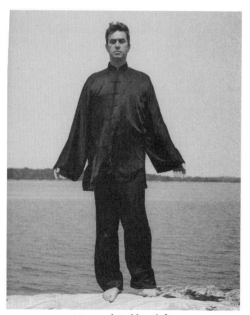

Hip and Ankles (left)

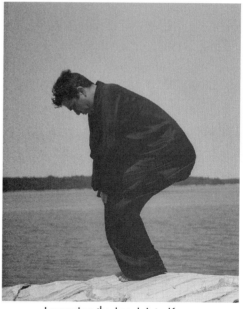

Loosening the Leg Joints–Knees

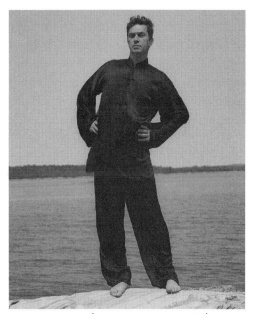

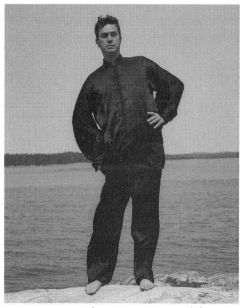

Loosening the Leg Joints – Hip (right)

Loosening the Leg Joints – Hip (left)

The tendons and ligaments in the legs are very strong, and working with them will quickly boost the entire body's energetic system. This is why we take time to give extra care and attention to loosening the legs, so that energy may flow smoothly.

START WITH 3 MINUTES, ONE AND A HALF MINUTES PER LEG, AND INCREASE YOUR TRAINING TIME GRADUALLY.

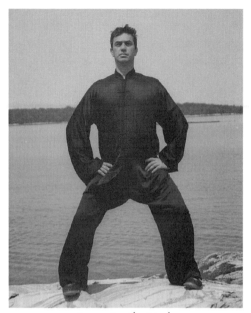

Loosening the Neck
(Center)

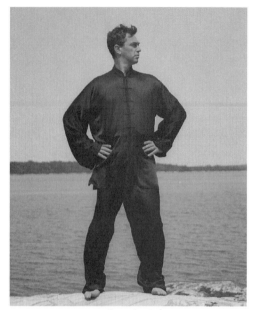

Look to the left

13. Loosening the Neck

Many people have different neck issues such as pain, or stiffness. To prevent stiffness of the neck, one must stretch the neck regularly, staying mindful of the its many muscles fibers. The neck has many angles and many ways of stretching, but these next few will give you a good start.

Look to the Left and Look to the Right

With your hands on your hips, inhale and turn your head to the left . Hold the neck where it feels it is being stretched for a few moments, then exhale and return to the center. Repeat this movement to the right. Practice this to the point where the muscle fibers you are working on become warm, meaning they have reached an excited state. Focus your mind in the area that is stretching.

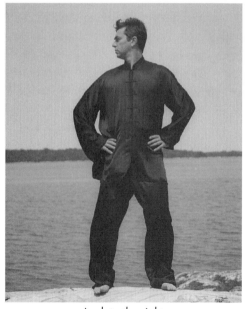

Look to the right

It may be too much tension for you to turn your neck if your arms are hanging down at your sides, depending on the flexibility of your neck. That is why I recommend that you start with putting your palms on your hips, which will keep the shoulders at the same height while you stretch the neck muscles.

While you stretch your neck, do not tilt your head or throw it forward. There is a tendency to do that in order to reach as far as you can. This is a shortcut your body and mind find to appear to stretch farther. Instead, make sure your chin is parallel to the floor and the face is not tilting to either side. Having a friend monitor you the first few times you practice this to verify your head is aligned is recommended.

The Pigeon Picks Up the Seeds

Move your head forward and down as if you were scooping up a seed from in front of you, and backward, in a circular motion.

Relax the jaw. Drop your shoulders. Relax the entire face. After a while, reverse the direction. Again, maintain a centerline through the head; do not tilt the head forward, backward, left, or right.

Around the World

The last neck exercise is for recovery. Simply rotate the head in small circles. Be careful when you roll across the back of the neck not to drop the head back too far. The vertebrae are not designed for the head to move back and rotate, and you will slowly grind your cartilage and discs away if you roll back too far. This is one of the common areas where most people develop arthritis in the neck. Rotate in each direction, without a grinding sound. If you hear grinding, make the circle smaller.

START BY STRETCHING THE NECK FOR ONE MINUTE PER EXERCISE AND INCREASE YOUR TRAINING TIME GRADUALLY.

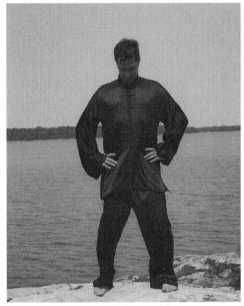

Around the World
(Down)

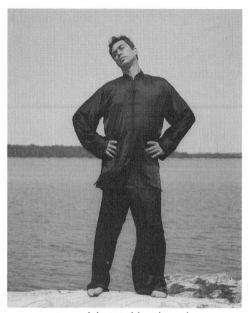

Around the World to the right

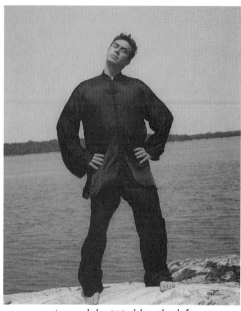

Around the World to the left

14. FLAMINGO STRETCH

This exercise combines strength, flexibility, and balance, which are essential for performing the Tai Chi movements, as well as improving your quality of life. Again, this exercise can be trained at a beginning level or at a more advanced level. Be sure the leg you are standing on has the toes pointing straight forward.

Place the foot of your other leg on a supporting surface, such as a chair. Be sure that your buttocks are even, parallel to the ground. There is a tendency to tilt, to collapse the standing leg's hip in order to perform this exercise. It is another shortcut the body finds to appear to be stretching farther. Drop the buttock of the standing leg and open up the hip joint.

To advance in this exercise, gradually raise the height of the supporting surface each time you train. Once your leg is raised all the way to your chest, wrap your arms around the leg, and practice this stretch without the chair while leaning against a wall. The advanced level of this exercise is to do it freestanding, squeezing the leg into the chest, and balancing on the standing leg.

This involves a combination of flexibility and balance. You are performing what your hip is designed to do. A main purpose of all of these exercises is to free your skeleton from being a prisoner of the soft tissue. The Flamingo Stretch offers an excellent

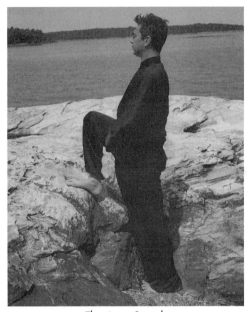

Flamingo Stretch
(Beginner)

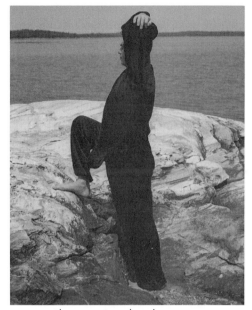

Flamingo Stretch with arms up
(Beginner)

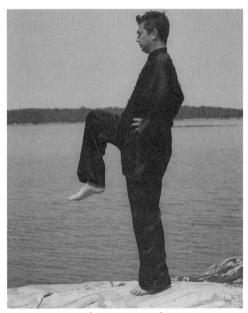

Flamingo Stretch
(Intermediate)

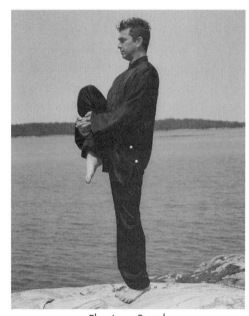

Flamingo Stretch
(Advanced)

opportunity to experience this. Usually when certain areas of the body are not able to stretch, it is because the soft tissue is shortened and is restricting the skeleton.

Once you slowly stretch and condition the muscles, freeing the soft tissue, you will be able to do what your body is potentially designed to do.

START WITH 3 MINUTES, AND INCREASE YOUR TRAINING TIME GRADUALLY.

15. SQUAT DOWN

Squatting down is beneficial for maintaining the range of motion in the ankles, which improves balance and prevents falls. It also protects the knees when done carefully, stretches the groin and lower back, and maintains a healthy digestive system. This physical ability will keep you young and able to reach the ground without injury.

For individuals with sensitive knee joints, monitor and protect the knees carefully. If this exercise is too challenging, hold on to something in front of you while squatting, such as a chair, to take some of the pressure off your knees. Increasing and maintaining the flexibility of your ankles is very important, especially for our purpose of performing Tai Chi. Stretching the ankles will allow you to move into deeper, more refined stances.

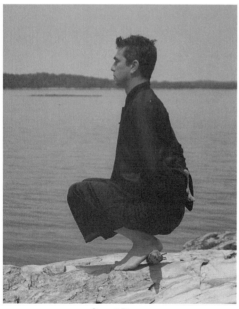

Squat Down
(Beginner)

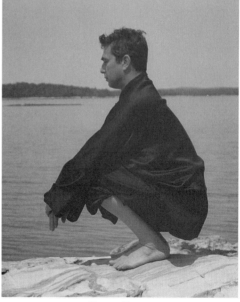

Squat Down
(Advanced)

Another purpose of stretching the ankles is to prevent falls at a later age. Having a larger range of motion in your ankles allows you to prevent falls in the future. Having a small range of motion in your ankle will make you stiffer, making you more susceptible to falls.

Again, this can be trained at various levels of difficulty. The first technique is for people whose ankles are not so flexible. Perform this stretch with the heels on something, making them higher than the toes, such as a board, or a yoga prop. Stay aware of tension in the knees and be careful. The ankle and knee area can take a long time to stretch, and it must be done gradually and consistently. Spread your legs the same width apart as your shoulders. Squat down while trying to maintain a straight spine. Remember to continue your deep breathing. Supply as much oxygen into the body as you can. This movement will also help your lower back, as well as having benefits for the digestive system.

Once you can do this comfortably, bring the feet closer to one another, and squat down, still using the height beneath the heels. Eventually you will be able to do this with the feet next to each other.

The next level of this training is to remove the height under the heels. Squat with the feet shoulder width apart. Then, after this is no longer difficult, again, bring the feet closer to one another, until they are touching.

The advanced level of this exercise is to squat with the feet together, toes pointing forward, and bring the arms behind your back, clasping your hands.

START WITH 3 MINUTES, AND INCREASE YOUR TRAINING TIME GRADUALLY. REMEMBER THAT THE LEG MUSCLES MUST BE ENGAGED. DO NOT COLLAPSE ALL OF YOUR WEIGHT ONTO YOUR KNEES AND ANKLES, AS THIS CAN CAUSE INJURY.

16. OUTER HIP

The next exercise will stretch the outer hips. Again, this is vital for performing deep Tai Chi stances. Flexing the ankle and the outer hip prevents injuries to the knees. This easy way of stretching the outer hip can be done at any time of your day when you sit with friends, or in front of the TV or the computer. Sit on a chair, with one leg in a 90-degree angle, with the foot flat on the floor in front of you. Cross your leg over the other, with the foot and ankle resting on the other side of your knee, the ankle of the crossed leg on top of the femur bone of the other. Using your hand or elbow, gently encourage the knee of the crossed leg to move down toward

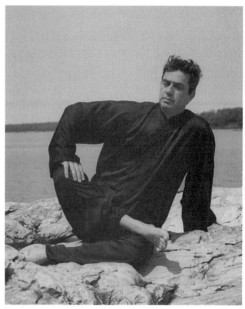

Outer Hip
(Beginner)

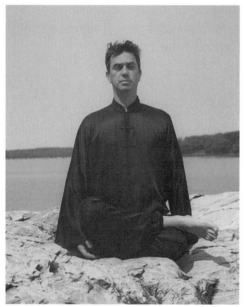

Outer Hip
(Intermediate)

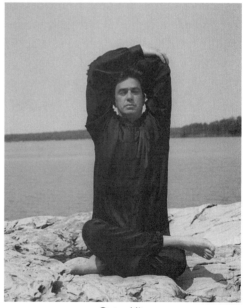

Outer Hip
(Advanced)

the floor. Sit up straight and breathe deep.

Maintain the visualization of the baton and sense the expansion from the center of gravity out through the skin, but also put your mind into the muscles that are being stretched.

A more advanced method is to sit on the floor. Again, cross one leg over the other, with the ankle of the crossed leg on the other side of the knee. Lean on the knee of the crossed leg and encourage it to move down. If the ankle of the crossed leg is too close to the leg it is sitting on, it may flex from the ankle, rather than isolating the hip area as we are trying to do.

Eventually, the knee will drop on to your other leg, and it can even reach the floor. Once you can reach the floor, you have very flexible outer hips.

Breathe deeply. Put your mind into any area of tension, and slowly dissolve it, while maintaining the energetic baton/bubble visualization.

START WITH 3 MINUTES, AND INCREASE YOUR TRAINING TIME GRADUALLY.

THE FOLLOWING THREE EXERCISES MAKE UP WHAT I CALL THE FIRE SET:

17. WALK AND KICK BACK

First Piece of the Fire Set

Remember to focus the mind and evoke your spirit throughout each exercise, and especially during these next three, which are the Fire Set of the preparation exercises. Your eyes should shine with a fiery spirit, as if you were in battle. In modern times, this warrior spirit can more often be utilized for raising the body's natural defense systems in the immune system, rather than engaging in combat.

This exercise will increase the heart rate, increase lung capacity, and strengthen circulation to get the blood to flow to the extremities, out to the surface of the skin, deep into the bone, and circulating smoothly through the organs.

In this exercise, you march in place, kicking the feet backwards as far you can. If you are very flexible, the foot can reach the buttocks during this movement. Put your hands on your waist and march!

Some days you can practice this slowly, some days you can speed it up. You may even do this at full speed, running in place. Be sure that you have loosened up first with other movements. Remember, keep breathing through the nose, and coordinate the abdominal muscles with the breath. Maintain the visualization of the baton. Keep the face relaxed and the spine straight. Deep, soft, quiet, inhalation.

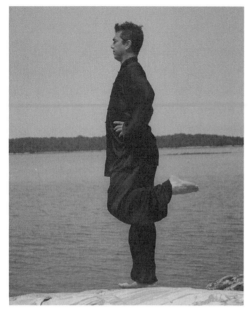

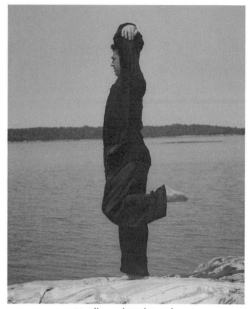

Walk and Kick Back
(Beginner)

Walk and Kick Back
(Advanced)

For a more advanced version of this exercise, which will also stretch the muscles around the lungs, put your hands over your head. This posture will be a little bit more challenging.

You will feel heat building up throughout the body. Remember, stop and close your eyes and then lead all of it into your energy centers when you are done.

START WITH 3 MINUTES, AND INCREASE YOUR TRAINING TIME GRADUALLY. DO NOT OVERDO IT.

18. WALK LIKE A WARRIOR

Second Piece of the Fire Set

This second exercise of the Fire Set, or cardiovascular set, for increasing your heart rate and oxygen intake is Walk Like a Warrior. It is similar to the previous exercise, except this time you bring your knees up as high as you can, emphasizing opposite arms with opposite legs. This can also get more advanced—the higher you lift the legs, and the faster you move.

Train the first two minutes just walking gently or lightly, and lifting the knees high. The higher you lift your knees, the more you demand from your heart, leg muscles, and lungs. Then, for one minute, run.

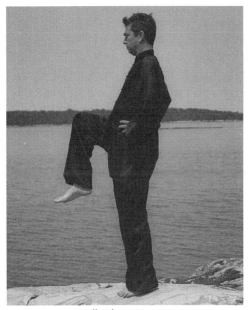

Walk Like a Warrior
(Beginner)

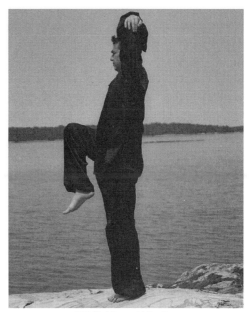

Walk Like a Warrior
(Advanced)

The reason I call this Walk Like a Warrior is so that students remember this is not only physical. I want you to literally sense as if you were running through a battlefield to save your family, or whatever it takes to evoke your spirit. The whole sensation of your body is like a warrior, with fiery eyes. You are in a fierce battle with yourself, against sickness, against feeling tired, or weak, or out of control. Take command of your health.

When you finish, surrender, and take the time to return all of this energy back to your center.

START WITH 3 MINUTES, AND INCREASE YOUR TRAINING TIME GRADUALLY. DO NOT OVERDO IT.

19. UP LIKE SMOKE, DOWN LIKE A FEATHER

Third Piece of the Fire Set

The reason this next exercise or mind/body prescription is called Up Like Smoke, Down Like a Feather is because, eventually, you want to be able to have the spiritual sensation of a feather falling from the sky when you sink, and the sensation of smoke rising up from incense when you rise up. "Be" the feather, and "be" the smoke.

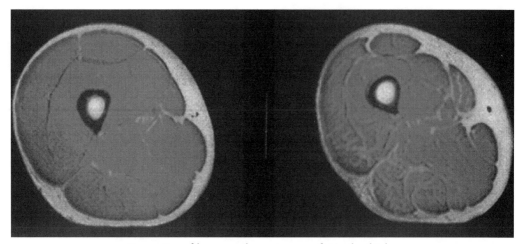

Proportion of lean muscle mass versus fat in the thigh.
Photo credit: *Biomarkers* by William Evans, Ph.D. and Irwin Rosenberg, M.D. (Page 54, Fig 2-3).

I designed this exercise after many years of experience working with martial artists as well as elders, and stumbling into many issues of leg strength, as well as osteoporosis and sarcopenia.

Osteoporosis is a condition in which the bones lose their strength and density. Sarcopenia is a lesser-known ailment. Another term for sarcopenia is vanishing flesh, meaning that you lose muscle mass, and that existing muscle mass becomes filled with deposits of fat. When you get on a scale, you are not aware that you have gained or lost any weight because your weight does not change. However, you notice the effects of sarcopenia in your daily performance. You suddenly cannot lift bags, you cannot open jars, your legs feel weak, and you do not understand why. What has happened is that your muscles have disappeared.

If you do not use it, you lose it. Muscle is replaced with deposits of fat, which does not give you the strength you need to perform your daily activities. When you lose independence because of issues such as osteoporosis or sarcopenia, you also have a tendency to become depressed, which inhibits your natural immune response to illness. It is a negative chain reaction.

In order to prevent these conditions, we can use physical resistance, using our own body weight. Studies done with sarcopenia and osteoporosis patients were done with common weight machines, free weights, cans, and resistance through lifting objects. I modified these exercises and created resistance by using our own body weight. It is just as if you are going to the gym and lifting your own body weight, again and again.

Up like Smoke, Down like a Feather will build muscle mass, stimulate bone growth, generate energy, and give you strong legs for a better quality of life, and for better Tai Chi.

In order to perform this mind/body prescription, you need to find a special place in your house, like a smooth wall, or the side of a door jam, or even the door itself. Just make sure that you lean against the door in the direction it closes, and not the opposite.

For the First Set, lean against the wall, and open your legs as wide as is comfortable; wider than your shoulders, if possible. For the Second Set, close the legs so they are touching. Once you have advanced with this training, you can go up and down on the balls of the feet, without the wall.

Throughout each stage of this exercise, your goal is to glide down slowly like a feather, and then float up like smoke. When you slide up and down, you do not want your knees to extended further than your toes. If the knees are further then your toes, you can easily hurt your knees. Place your toes out far enough that when you bend to where the thighs are at a 90 degree angle, the toes are still in front of the knees.

The next thing that can happen is when you come up; if your inner muscles are stronger than your quadriceps in the outer thigh, the knee will move in. The inner muscle will say, "Let me do it. Let me lift your weight up." What I want you to do is to think from your skeleton, from the bones. Do not let the soft tissue determine the action or the alignment. You decide to let the bones determine it and maintain alignment.

In the exercise, you will quickly find out which one of your muscles is stronger. Is it the inner thigh muscles or the outer thigh muscles? If your legs are together, and on the way up you want to open your legs then your quads are stronger. When the legs are apart, some people want to bring the knees in to come up. When the legs are together, some people want to open the knees and come up. The bottom line is that your body is going to rely on whichever muscle is stronger. We want to re-educate the soft tissues and make them balanced and have confidence that each one has its own individual strength and independence, rather than relying on groups of muscles that are not needed for that specific action.

Some people cannot even use the inner or outer leg muscles to rise up, and they use their hands to come up. This is okay just to get started, but what we want to do is bring back the strength and flexibility of our legs.

Remember, once you are comfortable with this movement, to maintain all the other internal skills while you are sliding up and down on the wall.

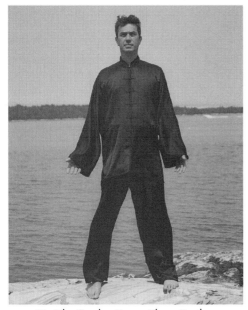

Up Like Smoke, Down Like a Feather
(Legs apart, Up)

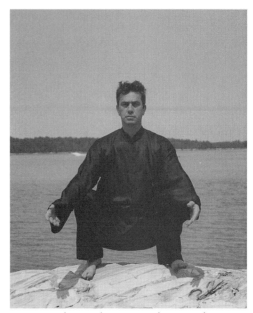

Up Like Smoke, Down Like a Feather
(Legs apart, Down)

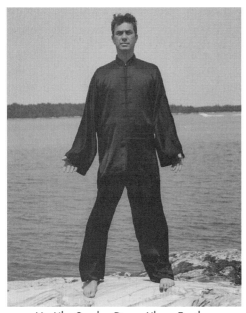

Up Like Smoke, Down Like a Feather
(Legs together, Up)

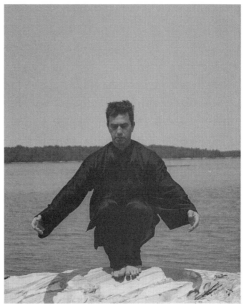

Up Like Smoke, Down Like a Feather
(Legs together, Down)

First Part of the Third Piece of the Fire Set

Place the feet about shoulder's width apart, and if you can go a little further, it is even better. The wider you open the legs, the more you affect the quadriceps, the outer muscles of the thighs. Slowly slide down and try to imitate a feather dropping from the sky. Then pause. Do not go further than 90 degrees.

On the way up, make sure the knees stay over the middle toes. If you need to, you may open the knees a little bit, and push gently up to rise like smoke.

Then slide down again slowly. Maintain your sacrum, or tailbone, touching the wall. Maintain the knees over the toes and push up. Try to coordinate your Center of Gravity breathing, maintaining the sensation of the baton internally, between the Upper Pituitary Gland and Lower Center of Gravity.

REPEAT AS MANY TIMES AS IS COMFORTABLE, AND GRADUALLY INCREASE THE REPETITIONS AS YOU CONDITION THE LEGS.

Second Part of the Third Piece of the Fire Set

Put your feet together. Maintain the same distance of your heels from the wall. Usually it is the distance between the knee and the sacrum. Another way of judging it is when you go down, the toes are still extended slightly farther than the knees.

Then on the way up, make sure that you do not open the knees. Sometimes the knees will want to open up to rely on the quads. Do not let them. You are in control of which muscles to use. Train this just like the first set, gradually increasing the number of repetitions. Try to train so that the inner and outer leg muscles are balanced.

Once you are more advanced, you do not need the wall any more. The problem is that when training this without the wall, people tend to come up with their sacrum sticking out. This causes you to divert your weight from being directly aligned above the legs, and you lose all the weight resistance in the legs.

Once you have trained on the wall until your legs are strong and the ankles are flexible, then you can practice away from the wall as long as you can keep the sacrum dropped. Again, train both sets, with the legs open, and then closed, slowly adding repetitions.

Using the wall is a pure way to isolate the resistance into the desired soft tissue. To transition from using the wall to free standing, you can hold the doorknobs of a door and gently support yourself, without hanging on to it, while maintaining the tailbone in, and then float down like a feather and rise up like smoke.

START WITH TRYING TO DO 50 REPETITIONS WITH THE LEGS OPEN, AND 50 WITH THE LEGS CLOSED, AND INCREASE YOUR TRAINING TIME GRADUALLY. IF THIS IS TOO CHALLENGING AT FIRST, DO FEWER REPS, BUT BE SURE THAT THE INNER AND OUTER LEG MUSCLES GET AN EQUAL WORKOUT. AGAIN, BE CAREFUL NOT TO OVERDO IT.

20. CRANE LIFTS TO HEAVEN

This exercise will cool down the body. Keep a healthy, upright body posture. Stay connected from the soles of the feet to the tips of the fingers, like the quiet, peaceful waves of the ocean. Evoke your spirit and sense as if you are a beautiful bird rising into the sky.

In this exercise, we will coordinate strengthening the ankles and calf muscles with the breathe and with stretching the two main bows of the body: the spine bow and the chest bow.

As we go up on the ball of the foot, we also release the bows, slightly bending the back, and moving our "wings" behind us. Then as we move back to the heels, we stretch the bow and raise our "wings" in front of us.

You may start training this movement standing in front of a wall, which psychologically, for some reason, helps you to reach a little higher with the ankles and the calf muscles, as your fingertips make contact with the wall behind you.

START WITH 3 MINUTES, AND INCREASE YOUR TRAINING TIME GRADUALLY. RELAX.

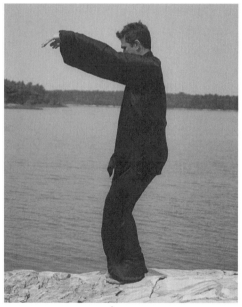

Crane Lifts to Heaven
(Arms forward)

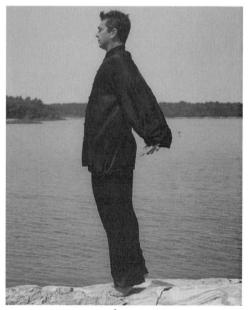

Crane Lifts to Heaven
(Arms backward)

21. SUN NOURISHING

Nourishing our whole being using the morning sun, during sunrise, is an ancient practice that was and is still trained by many individuals. The best way to achieve maximum benefits from this practice is to wake up thirty to forty minutes before sunrise and to wash up, and then drink warm tea or miso soup to warm the insides. Then, spend fifteen minutes warming up your body and breath. About five to ten minutes before sunrise, stand with your feet parallel, hip-width apart, and face the rising sun.

The practice involves directing your Third Eye area toward the rising sun and leading this energy in through the Spiritual Valley and down the center of the body, following the baton, all the way down to your Center of Gravity Energy Center. Continue doing that for no more than fifteen to twenty minutes after sunrise.

This can also be done sitting on a chair inside the house because the energy that we are looking for is not blocked by the windows and walls. Of course, finding a beautiful spot outdoors for this ancient practice during sunrise will result in a much stronger spiritual experience, which can later be used when you are practicing indoors.

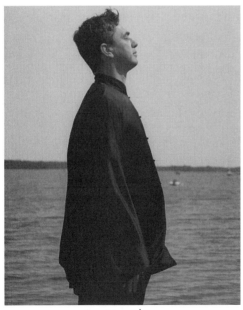

Sun Nourishing

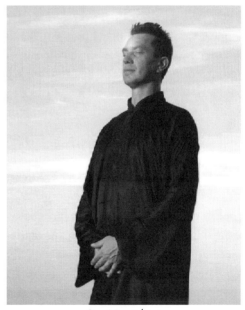

Sun Nourishing

To experience the nourishment more strongly when sitting, take a blanket and lay it on top of your legs and around your shoulders. Doing so keeps the energy inside the body and also creates the illusion every now and then, of your entire body consisting only of the trunk or torso. When standing, putting a blanket around the shoulders helps keep the energy inside the body and prevents its escape.

Positions for Practice

Stand outside ten to fifteen minutes before sunrise or sit on the edge of your bed. If you do not have a firm bed, I would recommend using a firm chair. A firm chair will help you lengthen the spine and create space for the internal organs. Sit on the edge of the chair so your spine is in this independent position. I like to refer to this posture as the Empress/Emperor position, because of the "lifted" feeling that sitting with good posture offers. You cannot rule your kingdom with a collapsed spine and spirit. We need to lengthen the spine. Mentally, the Emperor/Empress position also symbolizes a strong spirit. In this position, the eyes are strong, but not too intense. You must find the balance that symbolizes your spirit, which is between weak eyes and eyes that are too intense. If you feel fatigue in your lower back, there is another way of sitting. Support the lower back with a pillow or any object that will support but still allows you to lengthen the spine. When your back becomes stronger, you can alternate back and forth between the two postures—independent and supported.

Using a firm chair allows you to experience the lengthening of the spine more strongly. You also want to have your feet solidly on the ground in order to have a strong connection to the ground, to reduce stress on the joints, and enhance the connection of your energy with the earth energy. Lengthen your spine and imagine that your head is suspended by a thread from the heavens. Relax your shoulders. Gently, close your eyes and breathe deeply.

Steps of Practice

We are shallow breathers. From the moment we wake up in the morning, we should start stimulating the lungs, trying to bring as much oxygen as possible into the blood stream. Your lung capacity and oxygen intake will gradually improve over time. The more oxygen we can provide to our red blood cells, the better every cell in our body functions.

Breathe deeply through the nose. The tongue touches the roof of the mouth. Feel the ribs expand. Relax the entire face. Relax the corners of your eyes, the corners of your nose, the corners of your mouth, and let the temple area descend downward. Sense the entire skin of your face just melting. After you finish dissolving and melting the corners or the tight areas in the face, imagine the entire skin just melting down—layer by

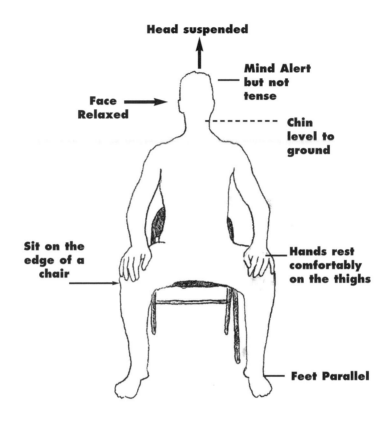

Stay alert but not tense; relaxed but not collapsed.
You are in command of your body and mind,
as though sitting confidently on a throne.

Emperor/Empress Position

layer, like an onion. Imagine you have ten layers in your face, and you just allow layer by layer to melt down, until you experience just the skull remaining.

Until you develop the habit of gentle, deep breathing, remember that we are shallow breathers. Breathe deeply.

Now, bring your mind to the Third Eye area, which is in the forehead between and in front of the two brain lobes, right behind the skull. When looking at a picture of the brain from above, you can see a split, or a valley, from the Third Eye area to the back of the lobes. This rift is referred to in *Qigong* as the Spiritual Valley.

Set your mind in the Third Eye and mentally lead the sun energy to this area. When holding the mind in the Third Eye area try, at the same time, to empty your mind from any thoughts. Maintain your focus on the Third Eye area.

Once you sense gentle warmth at the forehead, move your mind inward and down into the pituitary gland area, where the spinal cord connects to the two brain lobes. Another way to sense that area is by stretching an imaginary line from the the bottom of your nose and the bottom of the ears inward towards the center of your skull. This is the Pituitary Gland Energy Center, or Upper Energy Center. When you move the mind into the pituitary gland area, the sun energy nourishes the brain.

Make sure you breathe deeply. Make sure your head is suspended. Drop your shoulders. Relax the abdominal muscles. Then, slowly, move your mind down to the Center of Gravity Energy Center. After finding that area by stretching an imaginary straight line between two inches below the navel and the lumbar area, you reside in that centerline. Keep your mind down there, two inches below the navel.

When you are more comfortable and skilled with this complex visualization and energetic exercise of Sun Nourishing, you can also monitor the "Up and Down Forces." The Up and Down Forces are forces that exist within our physical body. You should develop the skill of being aware of them and emphasizing them, in order to help the body reach a deep level of relaxation and to allow the sun energy to spread throughout the entire body.

First, lengthen your lower back but do not push it into your stomach. We are looking to lengthen the lower back as opposed to collapsing it. This is an up force. Then balance this with the opposite, down force, by relaxing the abdominal muscles. There is a tendency to lift the spine using the abdominal muscles. Instead, I recommend that you keep training the back muscles and make them strong enough so that you do not have to use the abdominal muscles. The up force is the action of lifting the spine, while the down force is the simultaneous action of relaxing the abdomen.

The second up force is the thoracic spine. What you want to do is to bring the thoracic spine in and upward, as opposed to letting it collapse or straightening it too much like a military posture, which causes too much tension.

When you collapse your spine, you utilize only a third of your lungs, and lose two-thirds of your lung capacity. When you keep your spine straight and long, you are creating space for the organs and allowing more air to move in and more oxygen to nourish the entire body. By creating space for the organs, you make the organs happy. They are no longer compressed and stagnant.

In summary, creating space for the organs and the lungs, as well as reducing stress off of the vertebrae and the disks, are very important principles. Moreover, if you can continue using these skills throughout the day, your health will benefit tremendously.

Keep these main principles that we are looking for in mind: a firm base, lengthening of the spine, creating space for the organs and lungs, deep breathing to supply more oxygen to every cell, emptying the mind of any thoughts, monitoring the Up and Down Forces, and finally, leading the mind through the Third Eye into the pituitary gland area and down to the Center of Gravity Energy Center.

Your whole body is relaxed, but still contains enough force to hold it upright. Look for the motion in the stillness. Even though you are still, many things are moving—your breath, your thoughts, your heart, your diaphragm, your blood, and so forth. Try to notice what is moving while you are still during the time you are being filled with sun energy.

Sun Nourishing has many benefits, including developing the skills of deep relaxation, which in turn allows the body to use its energy for healing, and gives the immune system a boost. In general, it is just a very spiritual, comfortable exercise to do in the morning.

CHAPTER 4

Understanding Tai Chi Movements

"When being still, be still as a mountain,
When moving, move like a great river."

— *Wu, Yu-Hsiang*

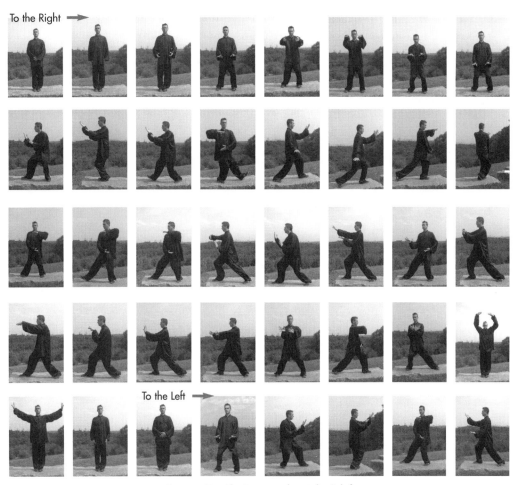

Sunrise Tai Chi Form to the right & left

BEFORE BEGINNING YOUR MOVING STANCES: TAI CHI DRILLS & FORM

Sacrum Dropped

If you want to achieve the maximum benefits from the mind/body program in this book and if you are interested in better health and the ability to generate more strength with minimum effort, alignment of the sacrum is essential. Because the sacrum is at the base of the spine, working on the sacrum will give you a starting point in achieving a larger goal, which is alignment of the spine as well as the entire skeletal system. Through correct alignment, we become directly connected to the earth and heaven. This is the fundamental first step on the path of achieving abundant energy through our bodies. At first, you will need to be more muscularly "active" to tuck the sacrum in using your abdominal and hip muscles, which will cause tension. Over time, however, as you become more flexible, you will be able to just drop the sacrum, using less force and generating less unwanted tension, especially if you practice the mind/body prescriptions described in this book.

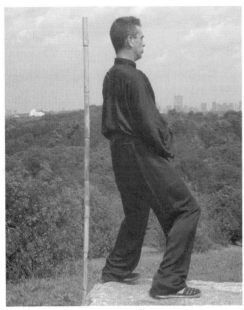

Sacrum Dropped (Correct)

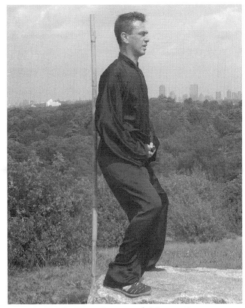

Sacrum Dropped (Correct)

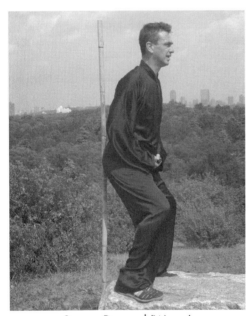

Sacrum Dropped (Wrong)

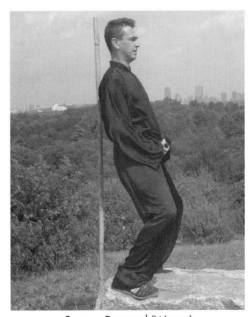

Sacrum Dropped (Wrong)

Head Suspended, Shoulders Dropped

We often allow our head to hang, and allow the neck to be compressed. We also have a tendency to have "floating" shoulders, and we hold tension in them and in the upper back. For these reasons, many individuals suffer from headache, migraine, and neck issues. In many instances, the shoulders are a major part of the problem, as well as the solution. The positions we sleep in for hours each night have a major influence on our neck and shoulders. Each one of us needs to find the best way to sleep without compressing the shoulders, or torquing the neck. The first step is awareness of correct alignment in the neck and shoulders at all times. Second are the mind/body prescriptions which give you tools to increase flexibility and strength in the upper body, from the solar plexus up.

In the East, head problems are not only addressed through the neck and the skull, but treatment includes the shoulders, as well as the chest and upper back. It is understood that there are thick, complex, and intertwined layers of soft tissue from the solar plexus area all the way up to the face. Your first step is learning the sensation of keeping the chin parallel to the floor. We tend to slouch and drop the head down, which puts it in misalignment. Some of us tend to tilt the head somewhat to the left or right, which again throws the alignment off.

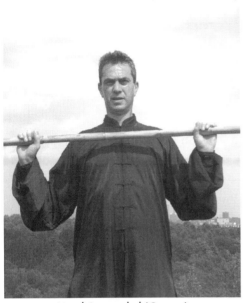

Head Suspended (Correct)

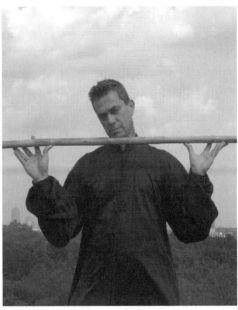

Head Suspended (Wrong)

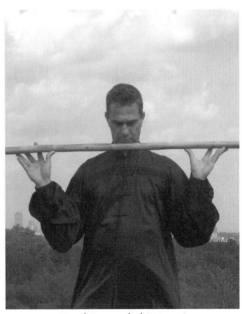

Head Suspended (Wrong)

Our shoulders are often misused. There are three common problems: We tend to have one shoulder higher than the other. We tend to "carry" one or both shoulders slightly forward which throws it out of correct alignment. Lastly, we tend to crunch or shrink the shoulders inward toward the neck, which can be associated with mentally holding tension in this area. Sometimes these behaviors happen because we do not use our shoulders much. If you do not use them correctly and regularly, you may lose their optimum alignment. Another reason is that we may sometimes suddenly abuse them or demand more than they can take while performing sports and hobbies, often after a sedentary period during which they can become weak and distorted.

Balance between strength and flexibility, and an understanding of alignment, are the key to having healthy shoulders, and pain-free neck and head. Some of the instructions that you hear again and again when learning the Chinese health or martial arts are: "Tuck your tailbone in, keep your chin parallel to the floor, lengthen the spine, drop your shoulders, and keep your head suspended." In the *Tai Chi Classics,* it is written: "Head held upright to let the spirit of vitality rise to the top of the head. Do not use external strength, or the neck will be stiff and the Qi and blood cannot flow through. It is necessary to have a natural and lively feeling. If the spirit cannot reach the top of the head, it cannot raise." Yang, Cheng-Fu (1883–1936)

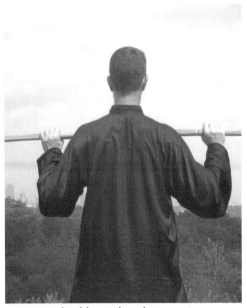

Shoulders Relaxed (Correct)

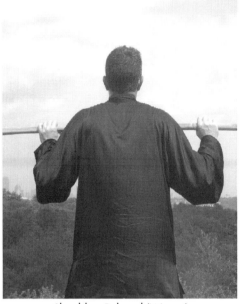

Shoulders Relaxed (Wrong)

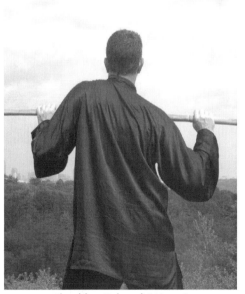

Shoulders Relaxed (Wrong)

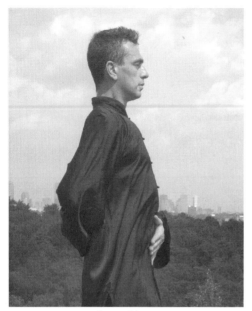

Empty Moon

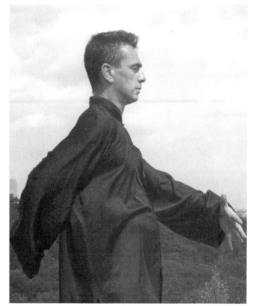

Full Moon

Empty/Full Moon

Physically, we want to regain control over our abdominal and back muscles. The muscles can move in or out on either inhalation or exhalation. When they move out, it is Full Moon, and when they move in, it is Empty Moon.

Elbows Dropped & Sunk

In order to have a strong flow of energy through the limbs, we should keep them slightly bent and sunk while performing all of the internal practices. One of the questions I was asked in the beginning of my mind/body journey by my teacher was, "If you needed to push up your weight onto an imaginary stone wall in front of you, using only your arms, what height would the wall need to be for you to push your weight off the ground with the least effort possible?" The answer is that the fence would need to be approximately the height of our navel, or belly button. Therefore, that is the position where we want to hold or keep our elbows when we do the Tai Chi drills or the Tai Chi form, with the hands at the height of the navel.

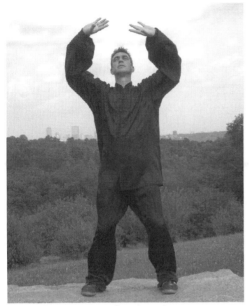

Elbows Dropped and Sunk (Correct)

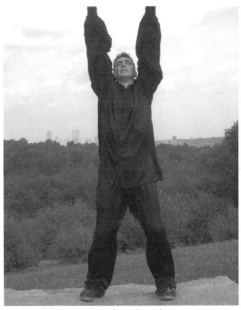

Elbows Dropped and Sunk (Wrong)

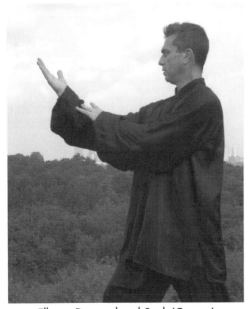

Elbows Dropped and Sunk (Correct)

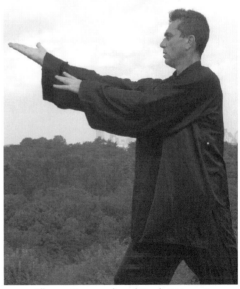

Elbows Dropped and Sunk (Wrong)

Weight Through the Knees and Not Into the Knees

We tend to misuse our knees, putting our entire body weight into the knees. Because the ligaments in the knees are not designed for that purpose, the pressure which accumulates in those ligaments is like a negative bank account. In this situation, many different problems can occur; some people gradually develop knee problems, such as persistent pain, and others end up with torn cartilage or meniscus, or hyper-extended ligaments, and eventually many end up with various types of arthritis in the knees. Our modern lifestyle often includes a lack of walking, climbing, and proper leg exercise, and a lack of weight-resistance through the legs. However, the biggest reason for so many knee problems is a lack of knowledge and attention toward correct alignment and not enough practice in the correct body mechanics during regular physical tasks. The knees are delicate; you must always pay attention to be careful with them.

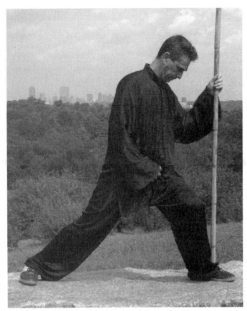

Front Stance (Correct)

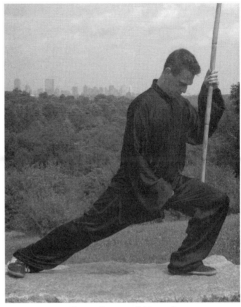

Front Stance (Wrong)

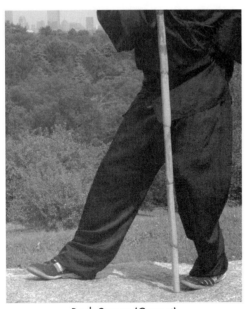

Back Stance (Correct)

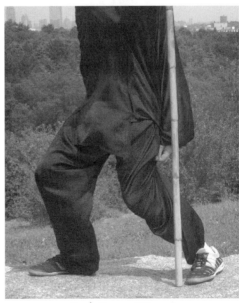

Back Stance (Wrong)

Turn & Lift Using the Heels

There are four simple rules regarding the feet, when lifting and placing the soles of the feet up and down, and when turning:

• When putting the leg down, start from the ball of the foot.
• Second, when lifting the foot up, "peel" it from the heel to the ball of the foot.
• Third, lift the legs and do not drag them.
• Lastly, when the foot is turning, it should have no weight on it, and you should turn on the heel.

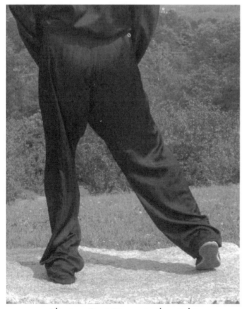

Placing Foot Down to the right

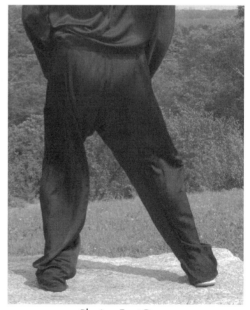

Placing Foot Down

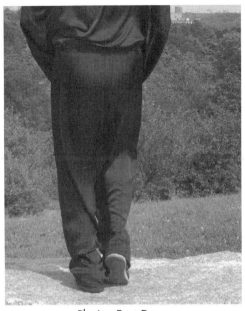

Placing Foot Down

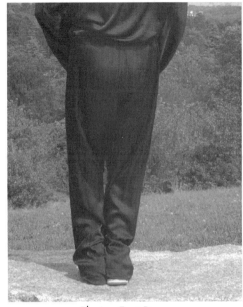

Placing Foot Down

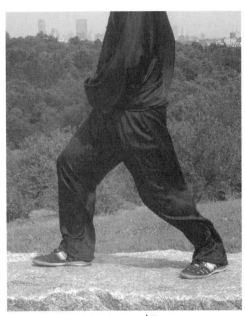

Emptying Leg and Turning

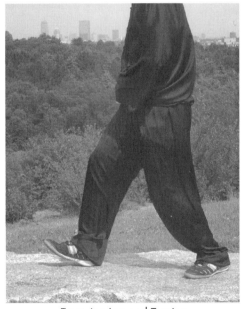

Emptying Leg and Turning

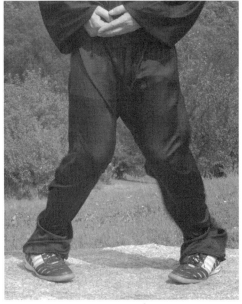

Emptying Leg and Turning

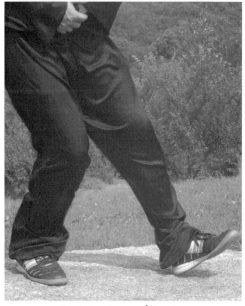

Emptying Leg and Turning

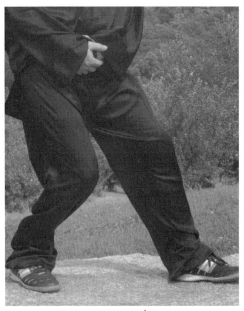

Emptying Leg and Turning

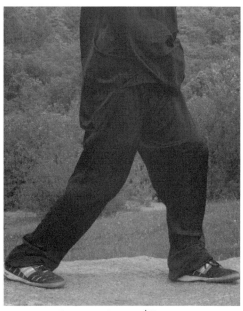

Emptying Leg and Turning

Tai Chi Hand Form

At this time, you should learn the Yang-style Tai Chi hand form. Using your left hand, start by slightly pushing the pinky sideways toward the left and the thumb sideways toward the right. The middle finger moves gently forward and up. Do the same with the right hand.

The reason that we hold our fingers in this manner is to create tension in the palm, creating a small dam, to slow down the energy that flows into the fingers and accumulate it in the center of the palm.

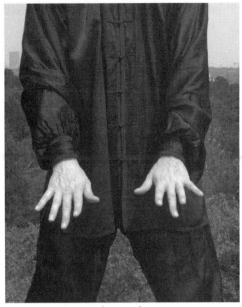

Tai Chi Hand Form

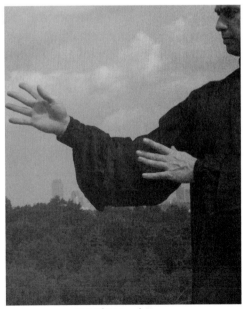

Tai Chi Hand Form

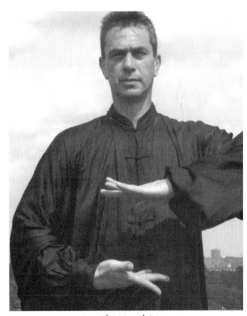

Tai Chi Hand Form

STANCES

Stances are the base of the Tai Chi form. You have to understand the stances, leg positions, and movements before you can perform a Tai Chi form. I teach my students to train the stances, the lower part of the body, first. You can also train only the upper part of the Tai Chi movements, such as doing the form while seated on the edge of the chair. This helps you to fine-tune the movements, and your Tai Chi will be improved when you put them back together. Remember, as we begin to move now into the Tai Chi postures and form, to maintain the skills and principles, both physical and mental, that we trained earlier.

Keypoints about the Stances

Each stance should be trained in a stationary position, and then you should train moving from one stance to the other. Remain relaxed, with a little bit of slack throughout the body, which allows the energy and blood to flow and nourish the body. Connect energetically to the ground. If there is too much tension in the muscles, the blood and the energy is stagnant and sealed, and your Tai Chi is not an internal art anymore; it is only an external form.

When you turn the body, be sure to turn the hips, and face them forward in the direction of the legs. Push off the heel of the back leg whenever you move forward. When you lift your foot at any time during the form, slowly "peel" it off the ground, or roll and lift it from the heel to the ball of the foot. When placing the foot down, "smear" it from the ball of the foot to the heel. Sense your body weight as it shifts from one leg to the other. Look for other differences throughout the entire body, as well.

Experience the substantial and insubstantial, which is the difference in levels of tension and relaxation, weight and lightness, in your legs, throughout your torso and the rest of your body. This internal sensing will raise your total body awareness. It is said in the *Tai Chi Classics*, "Substantial and insubstantial must be differentiated, not only in the legs, but in the entire body."

Mountain Stance

Stand with both feet together. Hands beside the body with the middle finger touching the middle of the outer thigh. Try to sense a high spirit; a connection to earth and heaven. Align the spine, drop the shoulders, and use deep Center of Gravity breathing. This stance can also be trained with your hands on your belly, to reinforce the sensation of the Lower Energy Center. You are a great mountain. You should be calm, quiet, and centered.

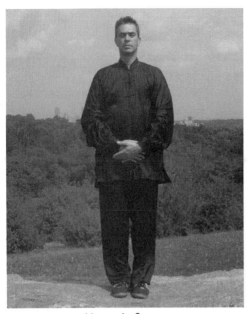

Mountain Stance
Eyes closed, palm on Lower Energy Center

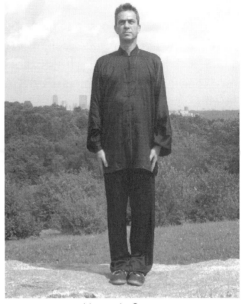

Mountain Stance
Eyes open, palms alongside the body

Begin Tai Chi Stance

From Mountain stance, step your left foot to the side, making your feet about shoulder width apart. Slightly bend the knees, but not too much. Keep the head suspended. Breathe deeply through the nose. The tongue touches the roof of the mouth. During exhalation, emphasize the sensation of the mind going out into the Four Gates, and on inhalation, back into your Lower Energy Center.

In traditional Tai Chi Chuan, this stance is called *Wuji* stance.

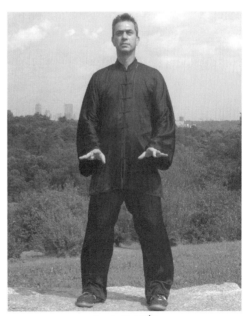

Begin Tai Chi

Horse Stance

Stand with the legs about shoulder width apart, feet pointing straight ahead, and squat down slightly. Horse stance is very common in all Chinese martial arts. In Horse stance, your squat can be as low as bringing the thighs parallel with the floor. In this Tai Chi form, you will not squat that low into Horse stance, but that can be an excellent additional training method for the thighs and entire body. You will experience Horse stance throughout the Sunrise Tai Chi form at various times, as you transition between the postures. The weight is evenly distributed, 50 percent in each leg.

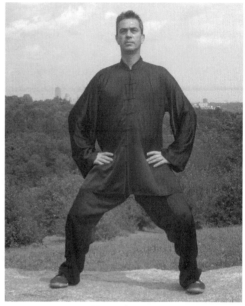

Horse Stance
50% – 50%

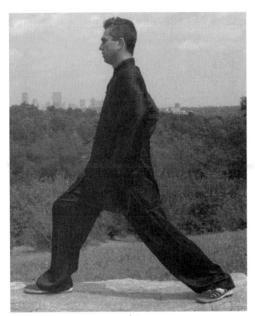

Forward Stance
70% – 30%

Forward Stance

Forward stance has 70 percent of the body weight on the front foot, and 30 percent on the back foot. The back leg is slightly bent. Do not bring your weight further forward than the toes. Your knee should not be further forward than the toes. The best indicator is the sensation that the weight is moving through the knee rather than into the knee. Direct your body weight through proper alignment of the leg into the ground. The toes should be turned 45 degrees. Make sure your legs are always at least shoulder width apart.

In traditional Tai Chi Chuan, this stance is called Mountain Climbing stance or Bow and Arrow stance.

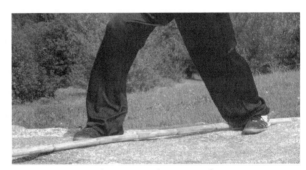

Forward Stance with correct alignment

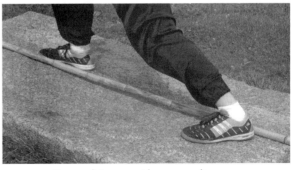

Forward Stance with correct alignment

Back Stance

Back stance has 60 percent of the body weight on the back, 40 percent on the front. The principles are the same as Forward stance. When you sink into the back leg, be sure to tuck the tailbone slightly in. Distribute the weight right into the floor, not your knee. You should maintain a solid connection to the ground with the soles of the feet.

In traditional Tai Chi Chuan, this stance is called Forty Percent-Sixty Percent stance. There are other traditional stances commonly used in longer Tai Chi Chuan forms, but these are the stances you will be learning for the Sunrise Tai Chi form.

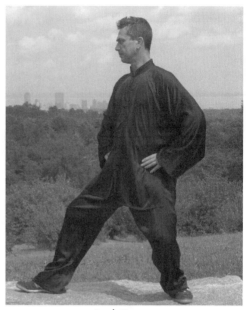

Back Stance
40% – 60%

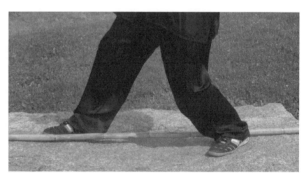

Back Stance with correct alignment

Empty Stance

Empty stance has 90 percent of your weight on the back leg and 10 percent weight on the front leg. The front leg gently touches the ground with the ball of the foot and is turned inward 45 degrees. It is important to distribute the weight of the back leg through the knee, down to the floor and mentally, you may go down even deeper into the ground, into your roots (30 inches deep).

This stance is also called Cat stance, which reflects the spirit that needs to be felt when holding this stance. First, start this stance standing high and as your legs become stronger drop the stance lower and lower while holding it for longer periods of time, 3 to 5 minutes on each side.

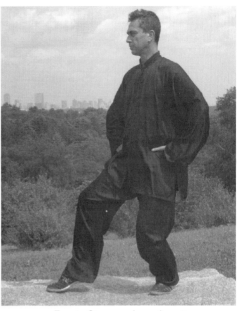

Empty Stance – Legs Apart
Waist turned away from the front leg

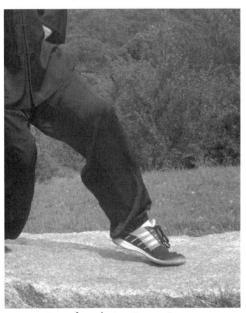

Front foot during Empty Stance
90% – 10%

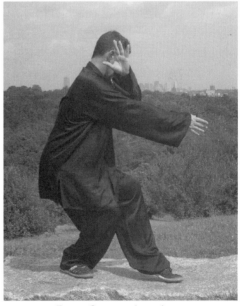

Empty Stance – Legs Apart
Waist turned towards the front leg

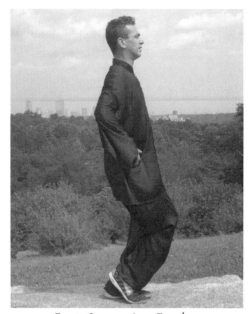

Empty Stance – Legs Together

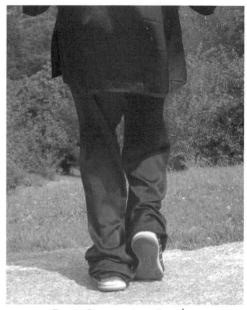

Empty Stance – Legs Together
90% – 10%

Make sure you do not injure your knees. First, develop balance between strength and flexibility in your legs before you require them to perform difficult tasks, such as low stances.

Your waist can be in one of two positions. At first, turn the waist away from the front leg, the leg with no weight. Then when you can keep your weight moving down through the back leg which holds the stance, you can move the waist toward the front leg, which has no weight. You will see that the second waist position in this stance is more difficult; both on the knee of the back leg, as well as on the lower back.

Tame the Tiger Stance

Stand in Horse stance with your feet parallel, sacrum tucked in, head suspended, and shoulders dropped. Put the center of your palms on your waist. On the next inhalation, focus your mind in the Lower Energy Center and on the sensation of 50 percent of your weight on each leg. Then, to begin shifting your weight, close your eyes and try to sense as if you were pouring your bodyweight like sand, moving from the left leg to the right, slowly, paying attention to the sensation of pouring the sand grain by grain.

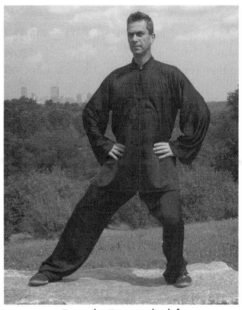

Tame the Tiger to the left

On the next exhalation, continue to shift your weight from the left leg to the right leg, ending with 80 percent of your weight on the right leg. Emphasize your weight moving down through the right knee into the floor and not into the knee. The left leg, which has 20 percent weight on it, is still parallel to the right leg. The inner soles of the feet are parallel to one another. You also want to keep both inner arches "alive" and engaged, especially on the left, because the action of shifting into the right leg tends to collapse the arch of the left foot, and vice versa.

I was told that this stance is called Tame the Tiger because when a tiger attacks you, the warrior waits until the last moment to respond. When the tiger jumps to attack, the warrior shifts weight to the side to evade the attack. Try to recreate the sensation or the spirit of the warrior when performing this stance. Shift your weight from side to side 20 to 30 times. Over time, you will be able to perform lower and longer stances.

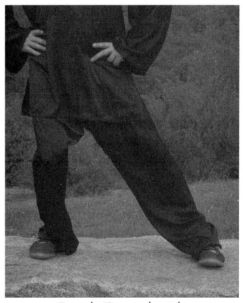

Tame the Tiger to the right

MOVING STANCES

Once you understand the stances and can perform them without thinking, you should start mixing them and move from one to the other while maintaining the internal visualizations. To make it easier, keep your eyes closed at first, and as your physical skills and mental skills improve, you can open your eyes. Make sure you understand the concept of leading weight through the knees, rather than into the knees. Remember that in order to prevent injuries and obtain the most out of the information presented in this book, the entire program needs to be practiced and used in a balanced way.

When practicing your stances, especially the moving ones, you have an excellent opportunity to experience substantial versus insubstantial in your legs first. Substantial and insubstantial are also known as *Yang* and *Yin*. When the weight is in the leg, it is substantial physically, but due to the increased muscular tension, it is insubstantial energetically. Tension creates energetic stagnation. Observe these differences during your stances, and as you shift your weight from one side to the other. An expert in the understanding of *Qigong* can go through ten levels of *Yin* and *Yang* when analyzing a posture or movement.

1) From Mountain Stance to Begin Tai Chi Stance

Stand in Mountain stance, center of your palms two inches below your navel over the Lower Energy Center, or with the middle fingers on the center of the sides of your legs in a straight line down from the hipbones. Breathe deeply when inhaling, focusing your mind in your Center of Gravity Energy Center, and upon exhalation, lead your mind down from your energy center through your legs, thirty inches below the soles of your feet. On the next inhalation, draw your mind up from the floor through your left leg to your energy center, shift your weight to your right leg, slightly sinking into that leg. On the next exhalation, move your left leg to the left, parallel to the right, and smear the sole of the foot gently on the ground, from the ball of the foot to the heel, without dragging the weight of the leg. The sole is about eight to twelve inches away from the right foot, or shoulder-width apart.

Leading with your mind, move your weight to the left leg until your weight is distributed evenly on both legs with your sacrum tucked in. Your mind is equally strong through both legs and into the earth below both of your feet. While you move your left leg, move your arms as well, with the palms facing down toward the floor, to the area two inches below your navel and with the elbows one fist away from the hipbones. Close your eyes

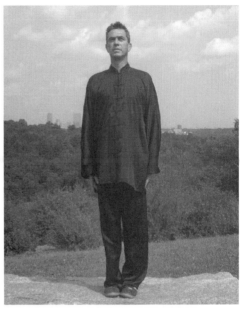

From Mountain Stance
to Begin Tai Chi to the left

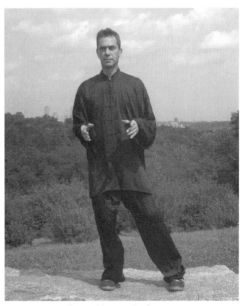

From Mountain Stance
to Begin Tai Chi to the left

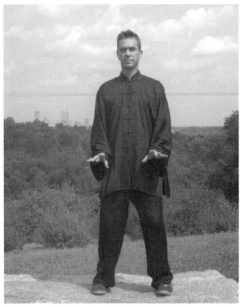

Begin Tai Chi

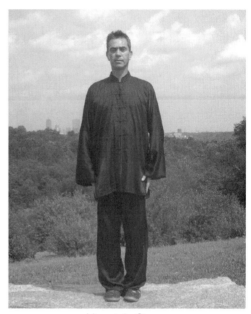

Mountain Stance

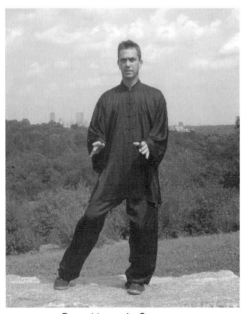

From Mountain Stance to
Begin Tai Chi Stance to the right

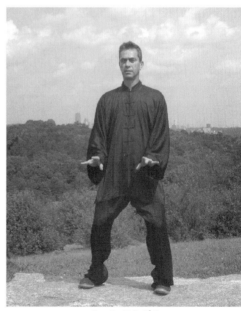

Begin Tai Chi

and practice Four Gates breathing and, if you can, add the baton/bubble visualization, as well. When your eyes are open, show strong intense eyes to raise the spirit. On the next inhalation, shift your weight to the left leg and draw your mind up through it. Pull the right foot, starting from the heel, and gently bring that foot back to Mountain stance. Bring your arms back to your Lower Energy Center or beside your legs.

Keep moving from one foot to the other, first in a straight line and then in any direction you desire. You should always finish Mountain stance with your feet parallel and palms gently on the sides of your legs. When you finish the Begin Tai Chi stance, your sacrum should be tucked in and the feet should be parallel to one another, knees slightly bent, elbows one fist away from the trunk, and with the palms facing down, two inches below your belly button. There is a tendency to have one foot turned to the outside, which is not the neutral position of your femur bone. The neutral position of your femur bone will line up correctly when the feet are parallel to one another.

2) From Horse Stance to Empty Stance

Stand in Horse stance, with 50 percent of your weight on each leg and put your palms on your waist. Close your eyes and visualize Four Gates breathing as well as the baton/bubble breathing. Shift your weight to the left without showing it externally, just enough that you can turn your right foot inward to 45 degrees. On the next inhalation, draw your mind from the floor through the left leg and shift the weight to the right leg, slightly bending the right knee and sinking your weight into it. Lift, but do not drag the left leg. Place the ball of your left foot gently on the ground without weight. Your weight should be 90 percent on your right foot with no weight on the left foot. Try to

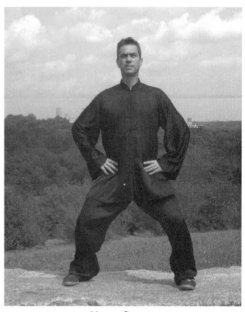

Horse Stance

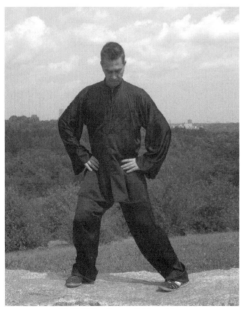

Shift Weight and Turn Foot

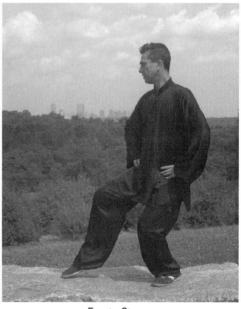

Empty Stance

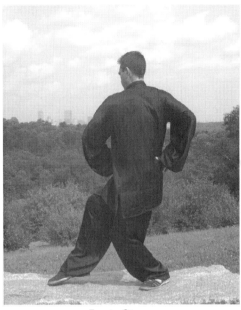

Empty Stance

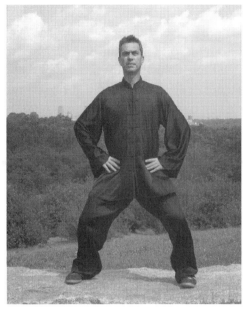

Horse Stance

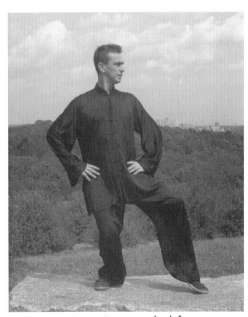

Empty Stance to the left

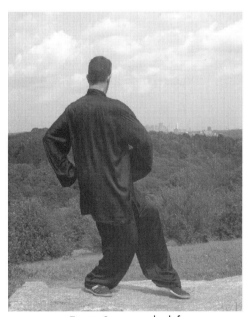

Empty Stance to the left

hold this stance for 30 seconds. As you progress, you will be able to crouch lower, and turn the waist more toward the left leg. Shift your weight back to the left foot and back to Horse stance.

Keep changing from side to side in a straight line. When your skill of these stances improves, you can turn and face any direction you desire while keeping the weight down through the knees, your head at the same height, hips straight forward, a 45 degree angle in the feet and about one to two inches between the toes of the front leg and the heels of the back leg. Remember when you are in Horse stance to keep your feet parallel, shoulder-width apart, drop your sacrum down, lengthen the spine, and maintain the internal visualizations.

When in Empty stance, keep both feet at 45 degrees with the sacrum tucked in and the weight distributed through the knees into the floor. The exercise "Up Like Smoke, Down Like a Feather" will help create the needed strength for these stances. To gain flexibility, work on the lower body stretches described in this program. To properly perform the Tai Chi form you will learn in this book, you will need to develop all these skills.

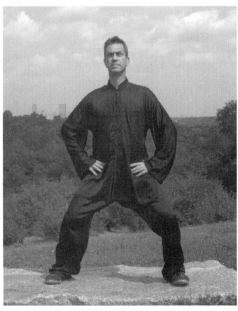

Horse Stance

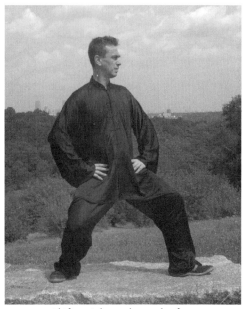

Shift weight and turn the foot

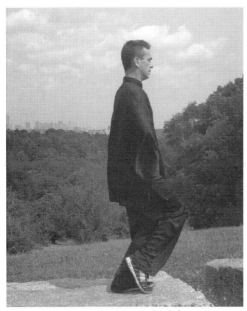

Empty Stance to the left

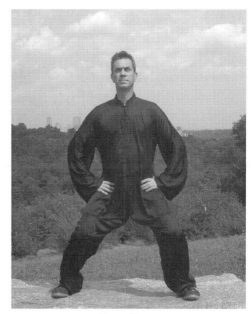

Horse Stance

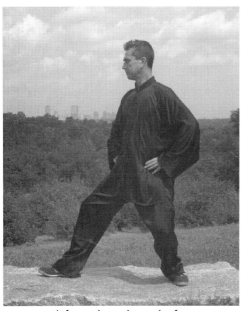

Shift weight and turn the foot

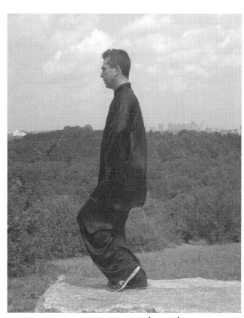

Empty Stance to the right

3) Forward Stance to Back Stance

Stand in Forward stance (Mountain Climbing Stance) with 70 percent of your weight on your right leg and 30 percent on the back left leg, with your feet set to 45 degrees. Turn your hips, pointing them straight ahead like the headlights of a car, toward the right. The back knee is slightly bent. You do not want to have your weight going into the front knee but rather through the properly aligned front knee into the ground. Place your hands on your waist or the center of your palms on your Lower Energy Center. The tongue touches the roof of the mouth.

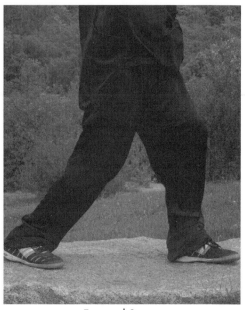

Forward Stance
30% – 70%

Close your eyes as you visualize Four Gates breathing as well as your baton/bubble visualization. When you are ready to move, on the next inhalation, gradually shift your weight to the rear (left) leg, and draw your mind up from the floor through the right leg into your Lower Energy Center and then down into the left leg as 70 percent of your weight settles into it, turning your waist toward the left leg.

Stay in Back stance for 30 seconds. Tuck the tailbone in, lengthen the spine, suspend the head, relax the face, and drop the shoulders. Continue breathing deeply. Coordinate the movement of the abdominal and back muscles with your breathing. Remember, when the muscles are drawn in we refer to it as Empty Moon, and when they are out, Full Moon. Maintain your internal visualizations. Push the outer edge of your left foot gently down against the floor. We have tendency to collapse the inner arches of the weighted leg, such as when we are in Back stance. The weight goes into the knees rather than the floor and that pulls on the inner arch, causing it to collapse.

We also tend to collapse the inner arches of the back leg when we are in Forward stance. Some of this is caused by lack of flexibility and some of it is just awareness. On your next inhalation, focus your mind in your Lower Energy Center, and on exhalation, shift your weight back to the right leg and lead your mind down through that leg all the way to the floor and beyond. Turn your waist toward the right leg so the hipbones are set straight forward.

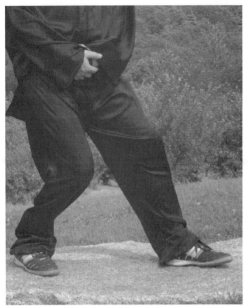

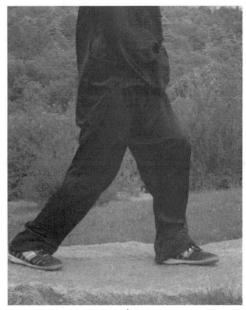

Back Stance on the right leg
60% – 40%

Forward Stance
30% – 70%

Practice moving from Back stance and Forward stance for 3 to 5 minutes on each side. The sacrum should be tucked in, the head suspended, and the shoulders dropped. Over time as your flexibility and strength improves, you can perform those stances lower and longer.

4) From Horse Stance to Tame the Tiger Stance to Empty Stance

Moving from Horse stance with your hands on your waist, shift your weight to your right leg, until you are in Tame the Tiger stance on the right leg. Move slowly, close your eyes, and experience a strong sensation of the *kua*, or the dome-like, powerful foundation of your legs. Once your weight is on your right leg, peel your left foot off the ground, starting with your heel. Then lift, not drag, the left leg and place it next to the right foot. You are now in Empty stance with 90 percent of the weight on your right leg. Roll the left foot down, starting from the ball of the foot, and shift your weight to the left leg. You are now in Empty stance with 90 percent of your weight on your left leg.

Now, empty your right leg, peeling the right leg off the ground, starting from the heel, and place it next to your right foot, from the ball of the foot to the heel. Now you are in Tame the Tiger stance with 80 percent of your weight on the left leg. Shift your weight slowly again to the right and stop when you are in Horse stance. Move about 10 times to the right and then 10 times to the left. Sometimes, you want to pause in between each stance for 30 to 60 seconds. During this time, close your eyes and visualize Four Gates breathing, as well as your baton/bubble visualization. This kind of training builds a strong experience of each stance, and it will make these stances and postures much better when you are performing the Tai Chi form.

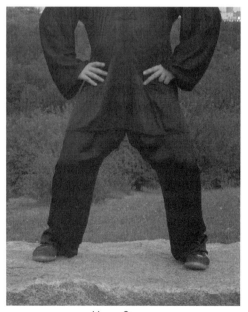

Horse Stance
50% – 50%

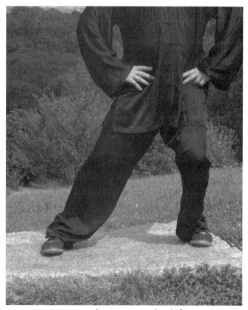

Tame the Tiger to the left

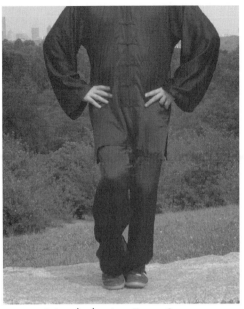

Bring the leg in – Empty Stance

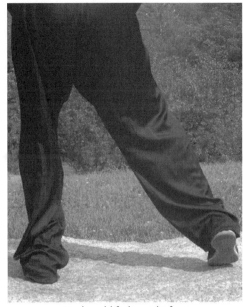

Peel and lift the right foot

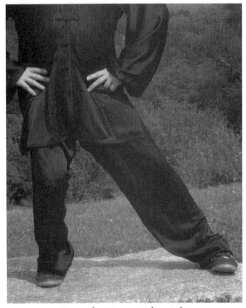

Tame the Tiger to the right

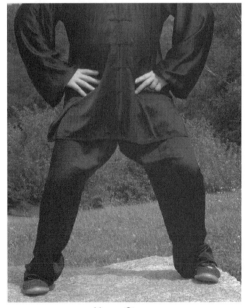

Horse Stance
50% – 50%

5) Forward Stance to Forward Stance

This time we will perform Forward stance from side to side. Start Forward stance with the right leg forward, hands on your waist, left leg back and the knee slightly bent. Push from the outer sole of the rear (left) foot and lead the weight through the right leg into the floor. Maintain your internal visualizations. The rule is that you can only turn the foot when there is no weight on it.

Starting by facing to the right. You will need to turn the right leg and foot 45 degrees inward. Because you have 70 percent weight on that leg, you need first to empty this leg just enough so you can turn the right sole of the foot on the heel. As soon as you empty the ball of your right foot, turn it inward so it is at a 45 degree angle. Then, pushing from the right foot, lift the left leg, continue the turning of the entire body to face the left, and then place the left leg down, slightly to the left of where it started, ball of the foot first. Repeat this change from side to side for 3 to 5 minutes.

You should always push off the back foot as you move into Forward stance, maintaining the connection of the body from the toes to the fingertips. Maintain proper alignment, posture, and distance between the feet. Keep practicing the mental skills. At first, you should empty the front leg completely and after turning the foot, fill it up again completely in order to experience the substantial and insubstantial through the body and especially in the legs. If you were to look at yourself from the side, you would look as if you are bobbing from side to side, left to right. This is acceptable, as this is only an exercise, but eventually you should refine the movement so that the weight shifting is not externally visible. In Tai Chi and *Qigong* practice, it is traditionally more proper for the movement to be smooth and continuous.

This exercise helps you to experience your body mass and to understand the substantial and the insubstantial aspects of the legs and the entire body. Through repeated practice, you can learn to smooth "corners" and stop bobbing from side to side. Experiencing the substantial and insubstantial in your legs is much easier than the rest of the body. This is why we start from the legs using big movements, such as bobbing in this case. As your sensitivity and awareness improves, smooth the "corners" and move in a straight line from left to right without bobbing.

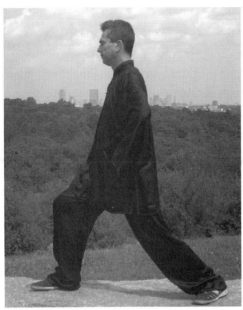

Forward Stance on the right leg
70% – 30%

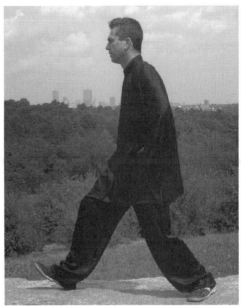

Shift weight and turn foot

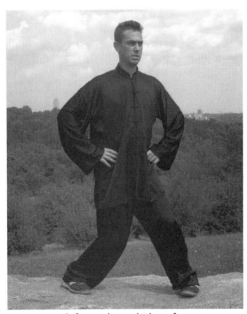

Shift weight and place foot

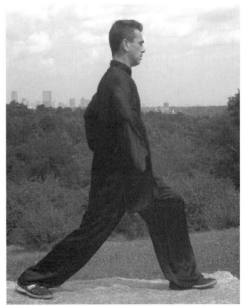

Forward Stance on the left leg
70% – 30%

6) From Back Stance to Back Stance

Stand in a Back stance with 60 percent of your weight on your back (left leg) and 40 percent on the front leg. Place your palms on your waist or on the Lower Energy Center. Make sure you distribute your weight through the knees into the floor, especially the back leg. Keep your head suspended, tailbone dropped, breathe deeply, and use Empty/Full Moon breathing, coordinating the abdominal and back muscles with your breath. Maintain your internal visualizations.

Your front (right) leg is already lighter because there is only 40 percent weight on it. Just turn the sole of the right leg inward to 45 degrees, then shift the weight to that leg while lifting the left leg outward and placing it down from the heel to the ball of the foot. Keep your waist at 45 degrees. Practice moving from side to side for 3 to 5 minutes. As you become stronger and more flexible, you will be able to move lower and perform the stance for longer periods of time.

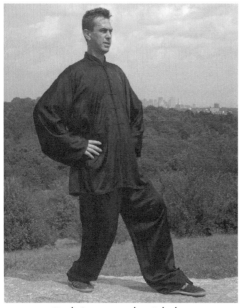

Back Stance on the right leg
60% – 40%

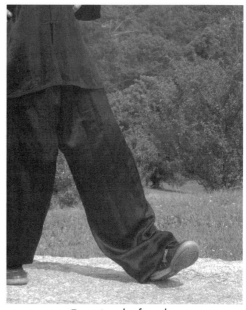

Emptying the front leg

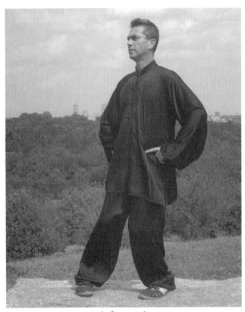

Shift weight

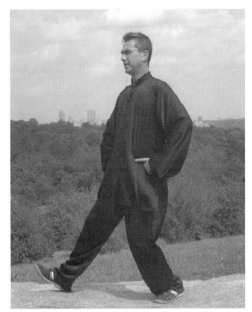

Place foot

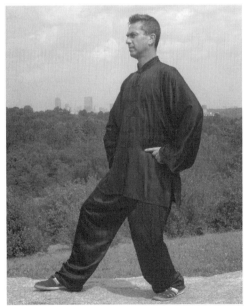

Back Stance on the left leg
60% – 40%

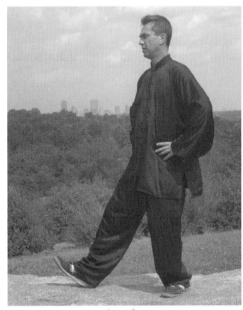

Place foot

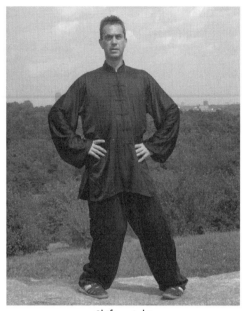

Shift weight

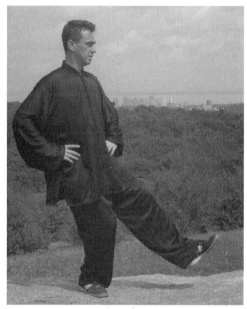

Place foot

STATIONARY TAI CHI MOVEMENTS—DRILLS

The Tai Chi stationary drills are designed not only for better health, but also to prepare you for the Tai Chi form. The stationary movements give you the opportunity to emphasize and experience the physical and mental skills more strongly when later doing the Tai Chi form. The drills also give you the opportunity to figure out how to put together the physical and the mental visualizations with movements from Yang-style Tai Chi. Each one of the Tai Chi movements you learn and perform have a martial application as well as specific benefits towards better health, longevity, and a higher quality of life.

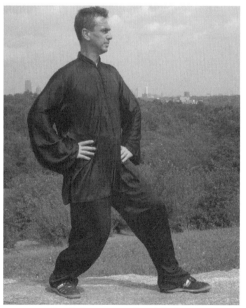

Back Stance on the right leg
60% – 40%

Remember the five building blocks: body, breath, mind, energy, and spirit. Try to bring all of them into the Tai Chi drills. The first part of each drill is stationary and the second part includes moving. As mentioned in the Tai Chi *Classics*, the whole body should be like pearls on a thread. If the movements are not a continuous, agile flow, the thread will rip and the pearls will fall.

To accomplish this concept of being one connected unit when moving takes time and practice. I recommend that you focus and emphasize specific skills from the different building blocks one at a time, and then at other times coordinate the skills with one another. For example, practice Grasp the Sparrow's Tail ten times while emphasizing the movement of the spine and chest bows. Focus on just stretching the bow and releasing it. Then practice the posture another ten times focusing on the skill of Empty/Full Moon breathing. Then, for the mental visualizations, practice ten times emphasizing only the Four Gates breathing. Again, ten more times, while just focusing on the baton/bubble visualization. Sometimes, I practice just my legs while putting the center of my palms two inches below the navel, and other times I sit on the edge of the chair and just focus on the upper body. When you are ready to practice the physical and the mental together, and include moving the bows, Empty/Full Moon, and Four Gates breathing, and the baton/bubble energetic visualization all at once, do the drills more slowly. You may find that closing your eyes at first will help.

Remember the sensation of the Tai Chi Ball exercise and try to recreate this sensation without the ball in your Four Gates breathing, as well as in your Upper and Lower Energy Centers. If you are flexible and your legs are strong, you will be able to perform the Tai Chi form with low stances, but when doing so, make sure you are not sacrificing correct physical alignment: sacrum tucked in, head suspended and shoulders dropped.

Protect your knees; your weight should go through the knees, not into them. Your mind should be in a deeply relaxed, meditative state, which is necessary for the internal visualizations. You should feel a strong sensation of the three forces, earth, human, and heaven. Strong abundant energy should be flowing throughout the body. Try always to smile when you practice, and carry the sensation inward to your mind, your chest, your heart, all your internal organs, and throughout your entire body.

1a) Grasp the Sparrow's Tail: Legs Stationary

Stand in Horse stance, arms raised slightly in front of you, with the palms facing down two inches below your navel, and your elbows a fist away from the body; this is the *Yang* part of the physical posture. Breathe deeply. Draw the abdominal muscles and the back muscles in and out with each breath. Bring your mind to the Four Gates on exhalation, and on inhalation bring it back into your Lower Energy Center. Add the baton/bubble visualization. On the next inhalation, stretch your bows, the spine and chest, drop the right elbow toward your body, and turn your waist to the right.

Maintain, through alignment, the open space between your inner legs, what is considered to be like a strong dome structure, which is referred to in Chinese as the *kua*. Now you are in the *Yin* part of the posture. On exhalation, push from the left leg and release the bows, emptying the abdomen, reaching with your fingers to your right upward in a 45 degree angle, and visualize grasping the tail of a sparrow. This part of the posture is again *Yang*. Using your Tai Chi hand form when extending to Grasp the Sparrow's Tail, lead your mind out to the Four Gates as well as to the bubble beyond the surface of the skin. When inhaling, lead the mind back to the Lower Energy Center as well as into the baton.

Next, bring the hand back to its original position in front of the body, by inhaling, stretching the bows, and drawing the right arm in. Exhale and release the bows while moving the arm down until your palms is two inches below your navel. Practice to the left and back to the center. Repeat 20 to 30 times to each side.

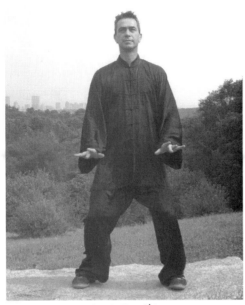

Begin Tai Chi

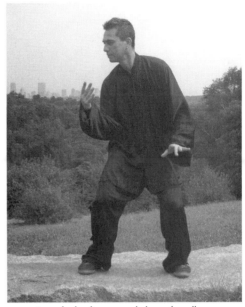

Stretch the bows and drop the elbow
to the right

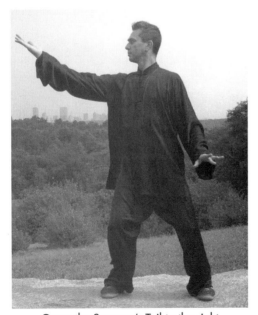

Grasp the Sparrow's Tail to the right

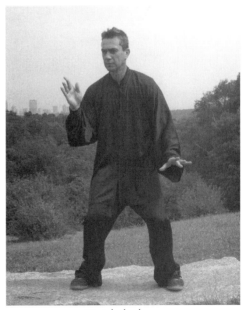

Stretch the bows

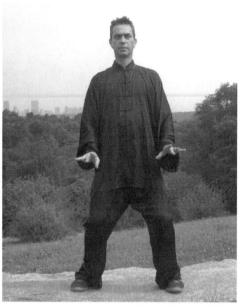

Begin Tai Chi

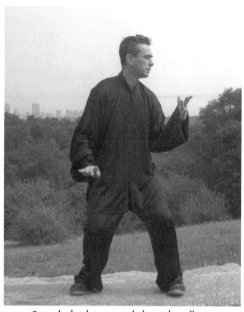

Stretch the bows and drop the elbow
to the left

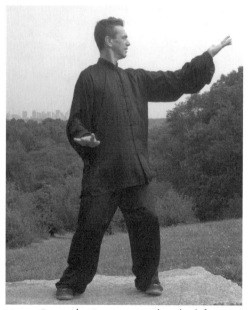

Grasp the Sparrow's Tail to the left

1b) Grasp the Sparrow's Tail: Legs Moving

This time we are going to do the same thing we did for the last movement, the only difference being that we are going to move from Horse stance to Empty stance, and back to Horse, both to the left and to the right. Once you drop the right elbow, shift your weight to the left foot, just enough so that you can turn the right foot on the heel toward the right 45 degrees. Push against the floor with your left leg and as you finish extending to Grasp the Sparrow's Tail, bring the left leg beside the right leg and keep it there with no weight, so it is just touching the ground with the ball of the foot.

Next, go back to the original position of Horse stance with the palms two inches below the navel. To do so, pull your left leg backward and stand in Front stance still facing the right. Shift your weight from your right leg to the rear (left) leg and turn your feet so they end up parallel and shoulder width apart. Do the same to the left side. Repeat 20 to 30 times on each side.

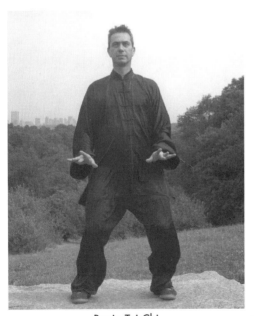

Begin Tai Chi

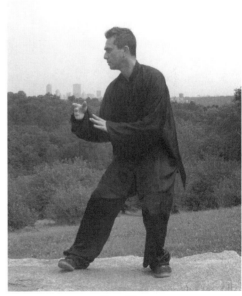

Transition

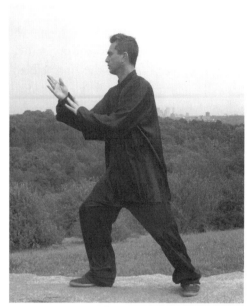

Transition

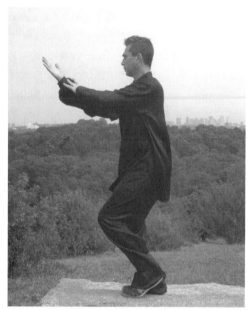

Grasp the Sparrow's Tail to the right

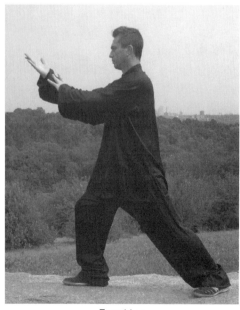

Transition

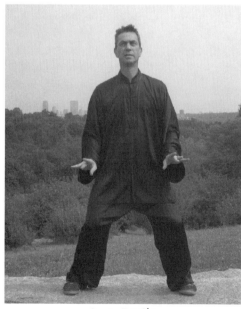

Begin Tai Chi

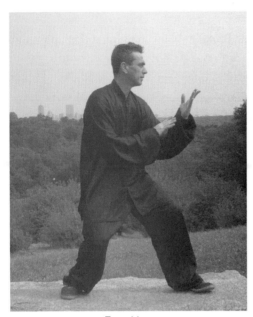

Transition

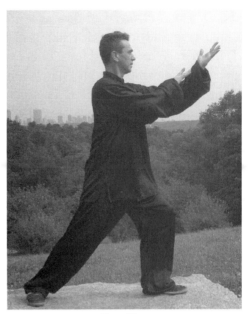

Transition

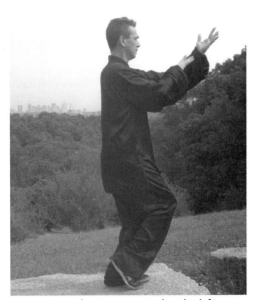

Grasp the Sparrow's Tail to the left

2a) Diagonal Flying: Legs Stationary

Diagonal Flying to left and right is similar in many ways to Grasp the Sparrow's Tail. First, get as low in Horse stance as you can comfortably practice, holding your palms facing each other and parallel to the ground, as if you were holding a ball in front of your internal baton. The right hand should be at the height of your navel and the left hand at the height of the solar plexus. Use your Tai Chi hand form.

On the next inhalation, lead your mind inward to the baton, and stretch your bows, tucking the tailbone in. On the next exhalation, push off the left foot and turn your waist to the right while releasing the bows. The hand that is on the bottom at navel height moves up from the navel diagonally to the right, fingers just above your head with the palm facing you like a mirror. Keep your eyes on that palm. At the same time, the left hand, which is at the height of the solar plexus, moves down and ends up two inches below the navel in the same position as in Begin Tai Chi, the elbow a fist away from the body with the palm facing down. It is as is you've torn or split the ball you were holding in half.

Then, turn the waist back toward the left and bring the right hand back to the solar plexus and turn it downward, while turning the left palm to face up, so that again you are holding a ball, except with the hands reversed. Repeat the same sequence on the left side. Maintain the space between your inner legs, the *kua*, drop your sacrum, suspend your head, relax the shoulders, and activate your visualizations. Repeat 20 to 30 times on each side.

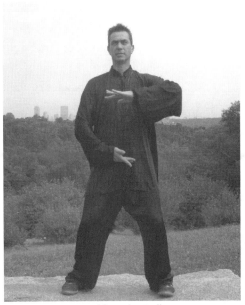

Holding the Ball
left hand on top

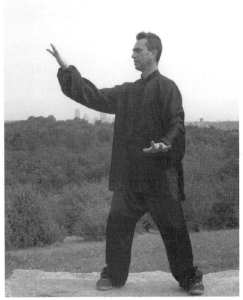

Diagonal Flying to the right

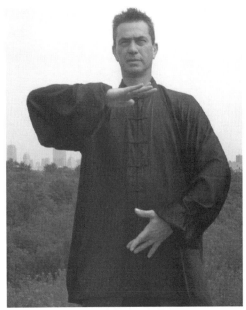

Holding the Ball
right hand on top

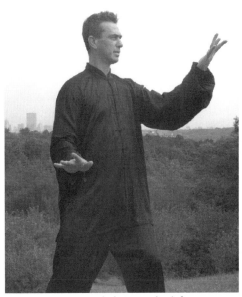

Diagonal Flying to the left

2b) Diagonal Flying: Legs Moving

Next, the upper body performs Diagonal Flying as before, and the lower body moves from Forward stance with the right leg forward to Back stance on the right leg. Then to the Forward stance on the other side with left leg forward, turning again to Back stance on the left leg, and then back to our starting position, the Forward stance with right leg forward.

Practice the stances first without the upper body. Once you feel comfortable add the upper body. When you are in a Forward stance, right leg forward, shift your weight back, into the left leg, just enough so that you can turn the right sole of the right foot inward to 45 degrees. Once you position that right foot, shift the weight back to that leg. Lift the left (rear) leg, place it slightly outward from its original position in a 45 degree angle.

At this point, you should be in a Back stance with 40 percent of your weight on the front (left) leg and 60 percent of your weight on your back (right) leg. Push from the back leg and turn your waist square forward, ending in Forward stance with 70 percent on the front (left) leg, and 30 percent on the back (right) leg. Remember to keep the correct distance between the toes of the front foot and the heel of the back foot. Keep the hipbones straight forward during Forward stance and at a 45 degree angle in Back stance. Tuck in or drop the tailbone down. The head is suspended, and the palms face each other at the *Yin* point of the physical movement. Repeat 20 to 30 times on each side.

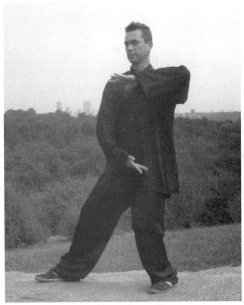

Holding the Ball
40% – 60%

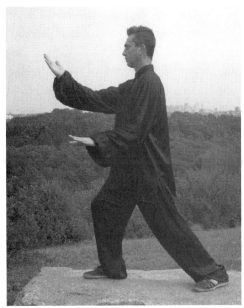

Diagonal Flying to the right

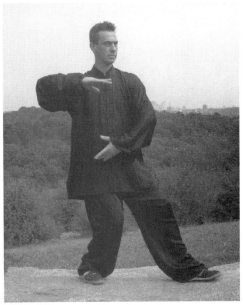

Holding the Ball
60% – 40%

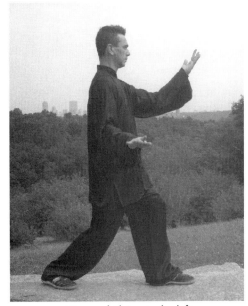

Diagonal Flying to the left

3a) Ward Off: Legs Stationary

While standing in Horse stance, imagine holding a big ball on your left side. The right hand is at the hip joint, facing up, and the left hand is at shoulder height facing down. The center of your palms are facing each other. I call this Ward Off stance, the *Yin* Ward Off. From *Yin* Ward Off, move to the *Yang* Ward Off. Move the right arm from your waist, upward diagonally, and stop when your palm reaches the height of the solar plexus. At the same time, your left arm moves down, as if you were pushing a ball down into the water and stops at waist height, directly in front of your navel; you are now in *Yang* Ward Off.

Another way to visualize *Yang* Ward Off is to imagine the right hand as if you are hugging somebody, and the left hand as if you were touching their belly button. Now move back to *Yin* Ward Off: drop the elbow of your right arm down and inward, and rotate the waist to the right so you end up holding a big beach ball on your right side, left palm at the right hipbone facing up. Continue to move from *Yang* Ward Off to *Yin* Ward Off and vice versa, and over time, add all of the physical and the mental skills. Repeat 20 to 30 times on each side.

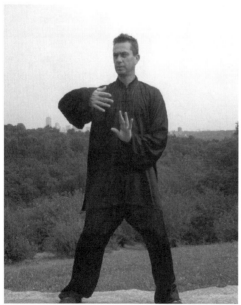
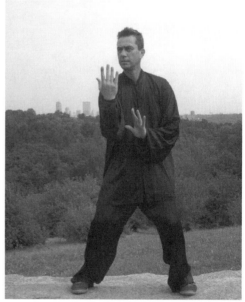

Ward Off to the right (Yang)   Stretch the bows and drop the elbow

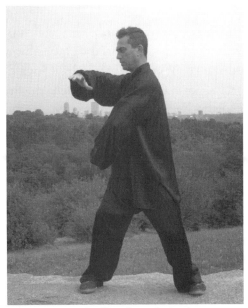

Ward Off to the right (Yin)

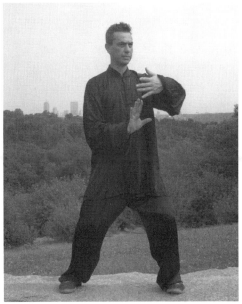

Ward Off to the left (Yang)

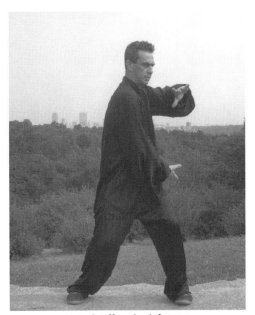

Ward Off to the left (Yin)

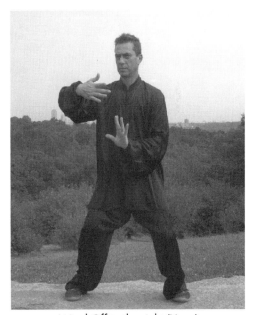

Ward Off to the right (Yang)

3b) Ward Off: Legs Moving

As before, practice your stances without the upper body and once you feel comfortable with the legs, add the upper body. During this drill, we need to move from the right side to the left starting with Forward stance. With your right leg forward, shift your weight to the right leg, move to the Empty stance with no weight on the left leg, and move your empty leg backward to the Forward stance, weight still on the right leg, which remains forward. Now, turn and face the left, emptying your weight from the right leg just enough so you can turn the sole of the foot on your heel. Once you have turned that foot 45 degrees to the left, shift the weight into the right leg. You are now in Back stance where your left leg is now the front leg with 40 percent of the weight on it, and the right is now the back leg.

Next, we move to Forward stance on the other leg with the left leg forward, and finish with Empty stance with no weight on the right leg. Keep moving from side to side until you feel comfortable. Remember, in the Forward stance, the hip bones are facing forward. Tuck the tailbone in. The head is suspended. Push into the outer edge of the feet. Use the bows and coordinate all of your skills with the in and out movement of your abdominal and back muscles or what we metaphorically refer to as Empty/Full Moon breathing. Power is generated from the floor, directed by the waist, and manifested in the fingers. Connect to the three forces. Repeat 20 to 30 times on each side.

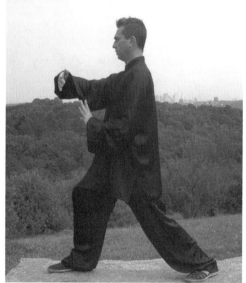

Ward Off to the right (Yang)

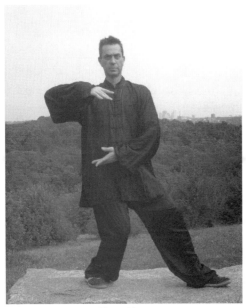

Transition

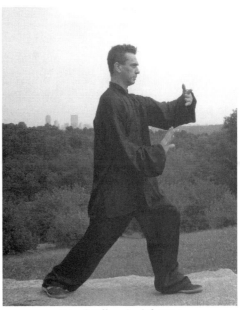

Ward Off to the left (Yin)

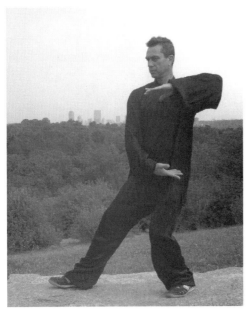

Transition

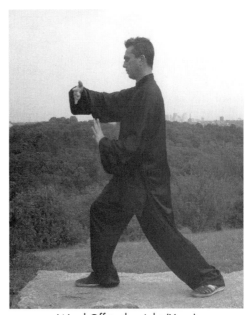

Ward Off to the right (Yang)

4a) Press: Legs Stationary

Stand with your feet together, as in Mountain stance, slightly bending the knees, and breathing deeply. We will be pressing forward, with the back of the wrist and the forearm, supported by the opposite hand. To start, put your left arm across your stomach, touching gently, and hold your left palm at your right waist, with the palm facing your body. Touch the inner wrist of the left arm with the palm of the right hand. At your next inhalation, bend the knees, "stretch" the spine and chest bows. Round the upper back, so if you were to see a side view of the body, it would look slightly curved, which is known in *Qigong* as Turtle Back.

Focus your spirit, and lead your mind to the baton. On the next exhalation, push from the ground, turn your waist slightly, "release" the bows, and press forward with your right arm pushing against the left wrist. Expand your mind to the Four Gates and the bubble. Do not straighten your elbows; always keep them slightly bent to allow the energy and blood to flow smoothly. On your next inhalation, bring your right arm across your stomach, and practice the other side; pushing forward with the outside of the right wrist and forearm. Repeat 20 to 30 times on each side.

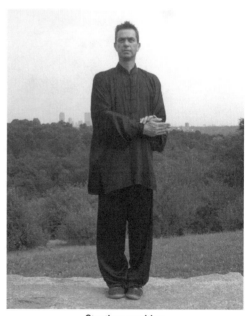

Starting position
Press at the left waist

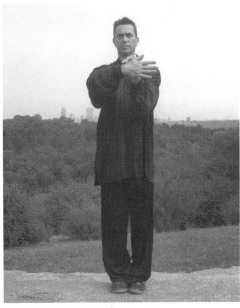

Press
Right hand in front

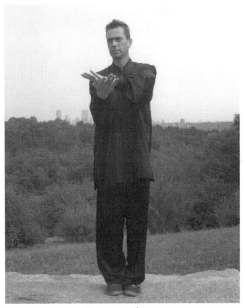

Rotate and turn

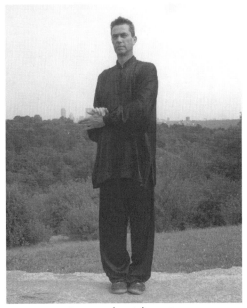

Press at the right waist

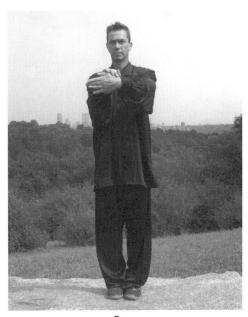

Press
Left hand in front

4b) Press: Legs Moving

Now we are going to Press to the right using Forward stance, right leg forward. Left palm touches the right wrist. Maintain your alignment; sacrum dropped, head suspended, and shoulders relaxed. This is the *Yang* part of the movement. Empty your front (right) leg, just enough so that you can turn the sole of the right foot on its heel inward to a 45 degree angle and shift your weight back into Back stance, turning the waist 45 degrees to the left. At the same time, change the position of the hands, rotating the palms in opposite directions, left counterclockwise and right clockwise with the wrists gently touching each other. This is the *Yin* part of the movement. Push from the back,

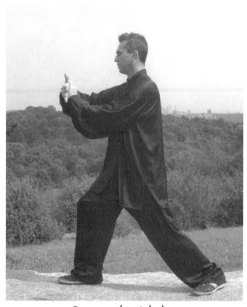

Press on the right leg
70% – 30%

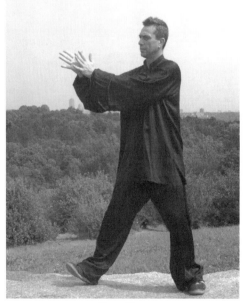

Transition

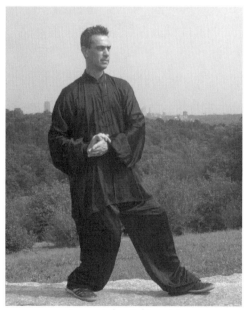

Press at the right waist

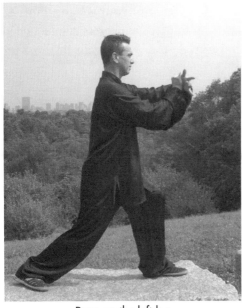

Press on the left leg
30% – 70%

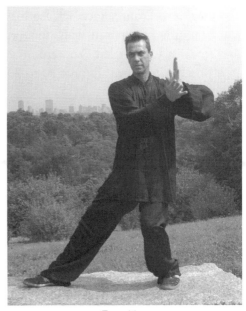

Transition

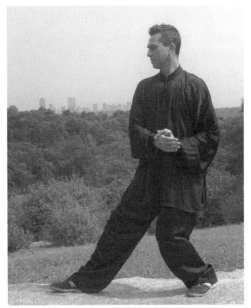

Press at the left waist

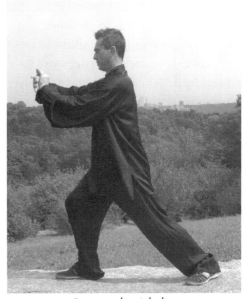

Press on the right leg
70% – 30%

right leg, into Front stance, left leg forward with 70 percent of your weight on it. At the same time, turn your waist forward, toward the left leg, and press the left wrist and forearm to your left. You are now Pushing to the other side, again in the *Yang* part of the movement. Repeat 20 to 30 times.

5a) Push: Legs Stationary

Stand in Forward stance, right leg forward, waist facing straight ahead, and head suspended. Hold your arms as if you were pushing a car, elbows bent and dropped, palms forward, and fingers pointing up. When we drop the elbows, we eliminate tension in the wrists, and create a stronger connection from the fingers to the feet, through the shoulders and back. The space between the arms should be the same as the space between your shoulders. Raise your spirit and gaze with fiery eyes.

On your next inhalation, sit back on the left leg and move your arms back like a wave that is breaking on the beach, keeping your waist straight forward. You should now be in Back stance, right leg forward and left leg behind, with your arms slightly closer to your body and fingers pointing straight forward. This is the *Yin* part of the movements. Do not fold, or collapse the arms too close to your body because for martial purposes, you will lose your strong structure, and for health purposes, the collapsed posture will slow down the flow of blood and energy.

On your next exhalation, push from your back (left) leg, and shift the weight forward to the right leg. At the same time, with your arms, push forward this time. You want to emit your power like a wave in the ocean lifting a boat. You should end up in Forward stance, right leg forward, arms forward, elbows dropped, and fingers pointed up. You are now in the *Yang* part of the movement.

Sit back and forth 20 to 30 times on each side. Make sure you distribute your weight through the knees and not into the knees. When performing the wave movements, try to lead the wave gently through the spine and the arms, as well as your wrists. To make the movement effective, you need to "be" the wave breaking on the beach when moving back, and "be" the wave lifting the boat when moving forward. Over time, you can add your other mental visualizations.

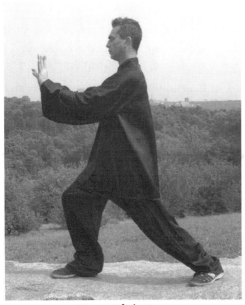

Waves Lift the Boat
Push on the right leg (Yang)

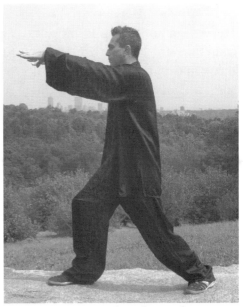

Waves Break on the Beach

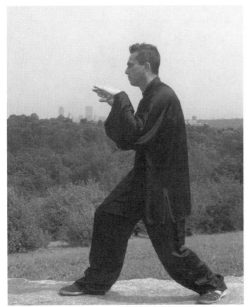

Push on the back leg (Yin)

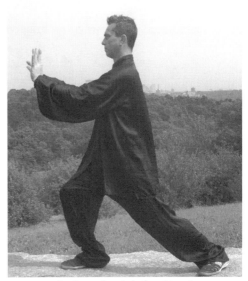

Push on the right leg (Yang)

5b) Push: Legs Moving

We are now going to move the wave from side to side, left and right, moving from Forward stance, right leg forward, to Back stance, right leg in the back. Make sure you turn the feet at least 45 degrees inward, so when you push off the right leg, and turn your waist to the left, there is no pull or torque on the right knee, and vice versa on the other side. When you are moving to Back stance, your spine and body emulates waves breaking on the beach and when moving to Forward stance, the body emulates waves lifting a boat.

This movement can be physically demanding. Development of your strength and flexibility is needed for performing this movement slowly in a low stance. Keeping your waist square forward, you should remember the wisdom passed on in the *Tai Chi Classics:* power must be generated from the floor, led through the legs, directed by the waist, and manifested in the fingers. Once you feel comfortable with the movement, add your other physical and mental skills, and increase the number of repetitions.

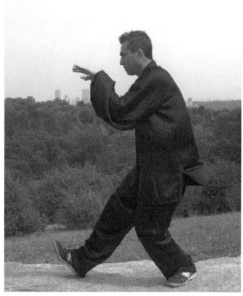

Begin Storing

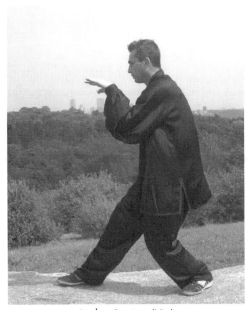

Push—Storing (Yin)

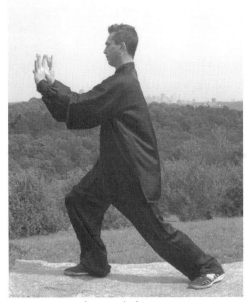

Push on right leg (Yang)

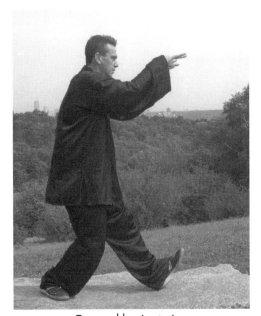

Turn and begin storing

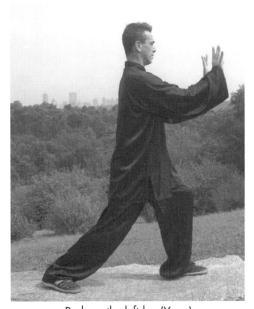

Push on the left leg (Yang)

6a) Single Whip: Legs Stationary

Stand in Horse stance and hold your left arm out to your right, across your chest, a fist away from the body. The right arm is extended out to your right. Bend both elbows and the palms face out, fingers toward the right. On the next exhalation, guiding with the waist, turn to the left, letting the arms follow, from your right to your left, like clouds moving in the wind. It is very important to maintain the dome between the inner legs by keeping the inner arches of the feet alive and the alignment through the hip and legs. The sacrum is dropped and the weight is distributed through the knees to the floor. Next, when you reach the left side, rotate the palms around clockwise to the left, with the elbows still slightly bent. Move like this from side to side 20 to 30 times. The waist turns, and the arms just follow.

6b) Single Whip: Legs Moving

We will now perform the same hand movements while moving from Forward stance, right leg forward, to Forward stance, left leg forward, turning on the heels. Maintain space between the toes of the front foot and the heels of the back when they are both in a 45-degree angle, so that your feet remain shoulder-width apart. Remember to maintain proper alignment through the skeleton. Relax, move the hands gently in the wind, and sense a softness through the soft tissue of the entire body. Switch from side to side, 20 or 30 times.

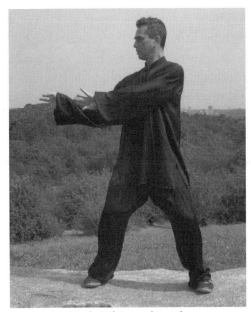

Single Whip on the right

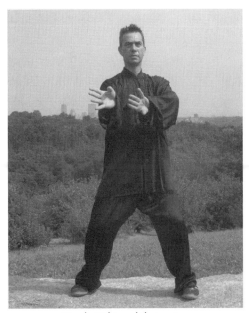

Single Whip while turning

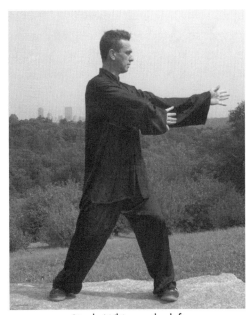

Single Whip on the left

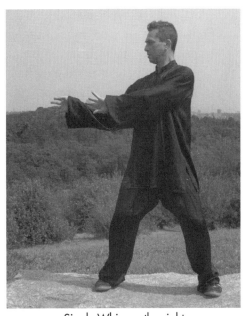

Single Whip on the right

WARD OFF, ROLLBACK, PRESS, & PUSH: LEGS STATIONARY

In order to experience the important energy patterns in the Sunrise Tai Chi form, I combined Ward Off, Rollback, Press, & Push into a set which you can be practiced on a chair, standing stationary or moving before learning the entire Tai Chi form. When performing this set stationary, we simply move from Back stance to Forward stance, back and forth, with correct alignment through the legs, to prevent injury and to experience a stronger flow of energy.

To help you memorize this set, the movements have been simplified and numbered.

One. Start in Forward stance, right leg forward, and hold the Yang Ward Off position. The right hand is as if hugging someone at the height of the ribs with the palm facing inward toward yourself. The left hand palm, fingers pointing up, touch the imaginary person's navel. Now you are in Ward Off posture.

Two. On your next inhalation, empty the ball of the right foot, "stretch" your spine and chest bows, and drop the right elbow toward the right hip, maintaining the space between your elbow and your body. The fingers of the left hand move next to the right elbow with the right palm facing you. This movement should make you feel like a cat right before jumping on its prey.

Three. On your next exhalation, push from your back (left) leg, and extend both arms forward and up in a 45 degree angle. Palms are facing each other.

Four. On your next inhalation, flip the arms so that the right palm is facing down and the left palm is facing up. The left fingers are near right elbow. Now, sit back on the left leg, exactly like pulling a rope backward to your left. Turn your waist to pull the rope. Now you are in Rollback posture.

Five. On your next inhalation, rotate your left palm, using the waist, so that the palm is facing down, and push from the back (left) leg to Forward stance, right leg forward. The left palm connects to the right wrist and presses to your right side. Now you are in Press posture.

Six. Change your hands into the beginning of the Push posture while still in Front stance, right leg forward. Fingers point forward, elbows are slightly bent, palms face down, and the center of left palm is over the center of right palm.

Seven. Sit back into Back stance while separating your arms; remember the waves breaking on the beach. Now you are in Push (Yin) posture.

Eight. Move forward and push; remember the waves lifting a boat. Now you are in Push (Yang) posture.

Over time you can perform the movements continuously, without relying on the numbers.

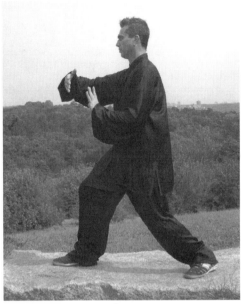

One
Ward Off to the right

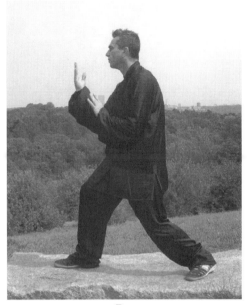

Two
Drop the right elbow

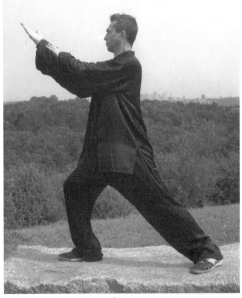

Three
Push and extend to the right

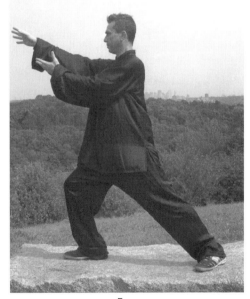

Four
Flip the arms to the left

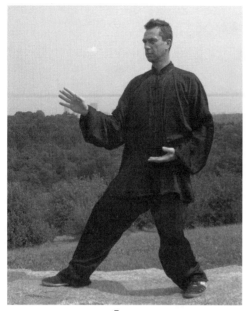

Four
Rollback to the left

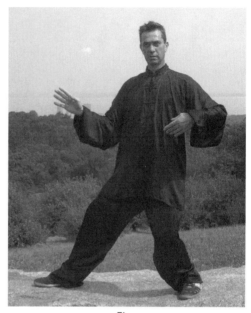

Five
Rotate Left Palm

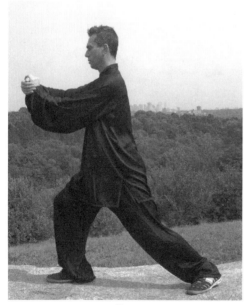

Five
Press on the right leg

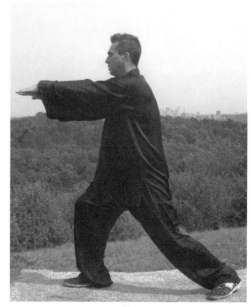

Six
Left over right

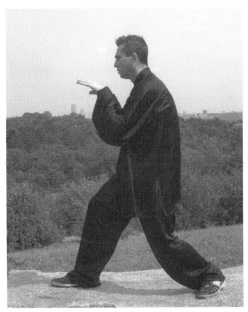

Seven
Sit Back on the left leg—Push (Yin)

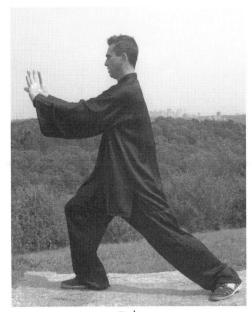

Eight
Push on the right leg (Yang)

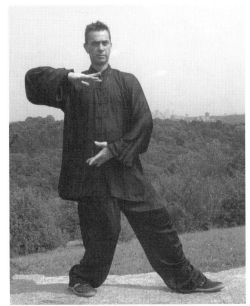

Transition from right to left

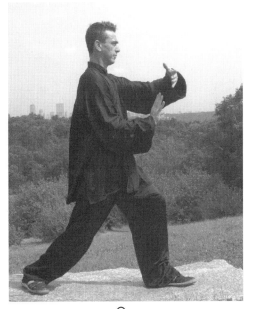

One
Ward Off to the left

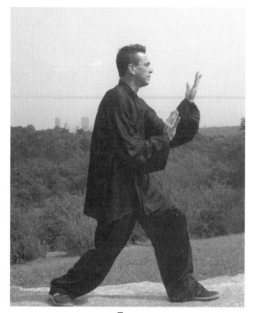

Two
Drop the elbow

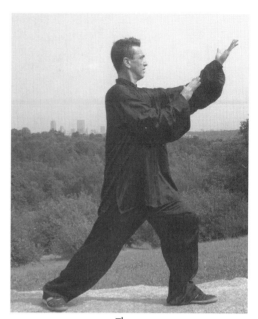

Three
Push and extend

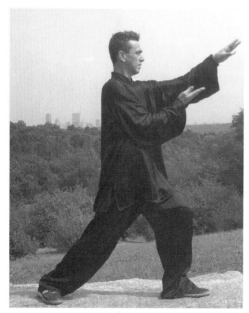

Four
Flip the arms

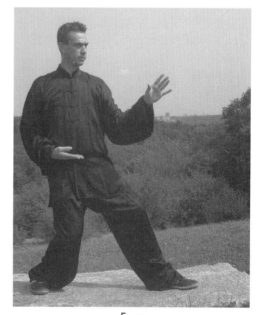

Four
Rollback to the right

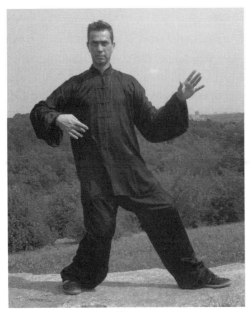

Five
Rotate right palm

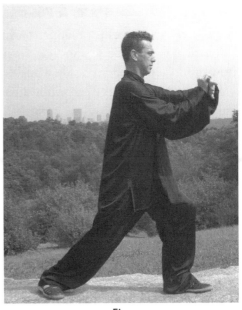

Five
Press on the left leg

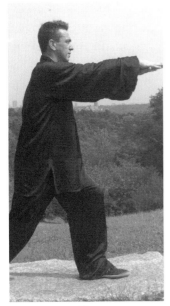

Six
Right over left

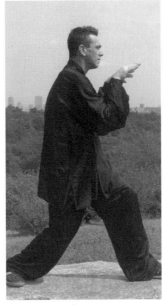

Seven
Sit back on the right leg –
Push (Yin)

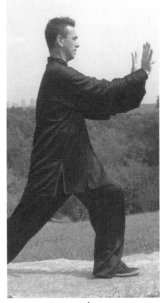

Eight
Push on the left leg (Yang)

WARD OFF, ROLLBACK, PRESS, & PUSH: LEGS MOVING

If you can perform the upper body movements comfortably while moving from Forward stance to Back stance, it is time to use what you have been learning until now to move from side to side while doing Ward Off, Rollback, Press, & Push. The sensation of each energy pattern is different and unique from one another: Ward Off energy feels like the body is a big ball bouncing off, or redirecting, any incoming force. Rollback energy is like a whirlpool; it is an energy that will twist, flip, suck, and pull you inward, and you can do nothing against it. Press energy is the sensation of two cars clashing head on. It is an energy that creates a strong squeeze or press.

Push energy has two parts; the first part, when moving backward, is like a wave that breaks on the beach—think of the massive waves in Hawaii. The second part, when moving forward, is like a wave lifting a boat in the middle of the ocean, as in the film *The Perfect Storm*. Remember, each one of those postures is an energy pattern, and each one of those postures needs to be trained over and over, until finally that pattern is experienced throughout your body, mind, and spirit to the degree that is entirely understood. At this stage you may begin to recognize those energy patterns, and others, in your surroundings, in your relationships, and throughout nature. We will discuss this in more depth in our next book, *Tai Chi Energy Patterns*.

Once you can perform the stances and movements from left to right, the next challenge is to perform the energy patterns in any direction, using all of the physical skills we have developed, while continuing to improve your focus on the "internal" aspects of the body, as well.

THE FIVE BUILDING BLOCKS

The Eastern arts divide our "being" into various elements, so we may better observe them as a whole. For example, yoga is sometimes symbolized using a triangle, which represents body, mind, and spirit. The philosophy of *Qigong* divides our "being" into five elements, which I refer to in this book as "the five building blocks of our being." These five blocks are: Body, Breath, Mind, Energy, and Spirit. Remember the five building blocks and try to apply them in each movement. Within each block there are a number of skills that need to be acquired.

When you are focusing on the Body block, emphasize the following: alignment of the skeleton, a softness of the soft tissues, Empty/Full Moon breathing, a "stretch" and "release" of the bows, the sacrum dropping, head suspended, shoulders dropping, face relaxing, and a gentle pulsing within the joints.

Within the Breath block: breathe long, deep, peaceful, quiet inhalations and exhalations. On exhalation, soften the muscles around the lungs. Move the air to different

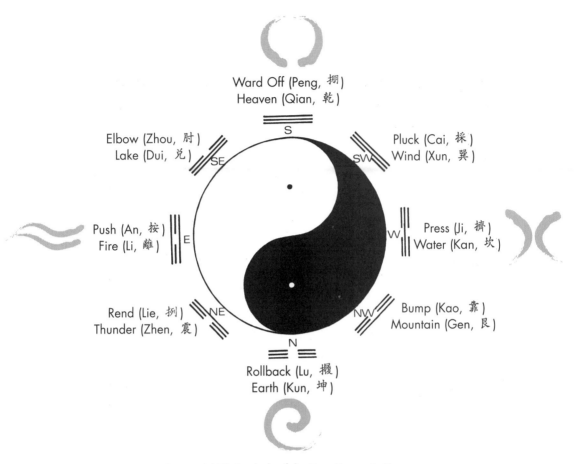

Figure 4-172 Symbols of the Four Energetic Patterns
(From Dr. Yang, Jwing Ming, *Tai Chi Theory and Martial Power*, p12, (YMAA Publication Center,1996)

parts of the lungs using the various postures which stretch the ribs and spine, which can be enhanced by moving the limbs and bending the torso. Pause briefly in the space at the end of your exhalation. This is considered to be the quietest time in our body.

In the Mind and Energy blocks, try to achieve a meditative mind—between awake and asleep. Spend time focusing on your internal visualizations: the baton, which you can visualize as having its lower ball in your belly, in your Center of Gravity Energy Center, connected by a line up to the upper ball in the pituitary gland area. Also, practice visualizing the bubble surrounding the body, or the Guardian Energy. Finally, work on leading the mind and energy to the Four Gates and beyond, and then back to your Lower Energy Center.

Regarding the Spirit block: learn each of Tai Chi movement's intent, and try to fulfill the "spirit" of each move. Develop the ability to "raise" or "cool" the spirit as needed.

Now you are ready for the Tai Chi form.

CHAPTER 5
Sunrise Tai Chi Form

On a physical level, the Tai Chi postures engage the whole body: The stances we have just learned utilize strength and flexibility, while maintaining or increasing the range of movement in the joints. The stances will increase muscle mass and bone density, which is important for health, as well as martial arts. The pulsing and pumping of the joints and ligaments boost our energetic circulatory system, the same system that we work on when we go to an acupuncturist.

Relaxing and tensing various groups of muscles creates a cycle of holding and releasing blood and energy into the veins and capillaries, as well as into the energy pathways, known as channels, vessels, and meridians. This works to open up and nourish the body's trillions of cells on the deepest level, all the way to the extremities. In a way, you are receiving acupuncture, or acupressure, and getting a Swedish massage at the same time, only through the Tai Chi movements.

The breath is used as a tool to quiet the mind and to lead energy in and out of the body. For martial applications, in general, when inhaling we block, and when exhaling, we strike. For health purposes, inhaling and exhaling is used for moving/leading energy to a desired area. This deep breathing brings more oxygen in, and more toxins, like carbon dioxide out, which upgrades the function of every cell in our body.

ELEMENTS OF THE SUNRISE TAI CHI FORM

To the left:
- *Mountain Stance*
- *Begin Tai Chi*
- *Grasp the Sparrow's Tail*
- *Diagonal Flying*
- *Ward Off*
- *Rollback, Press, Push*
- *Single Whip/Cleanse/Close Tai Chi*

To the right:
- *Mountain Stance*
- *Begin Tai Chi*
- *Grasp the Sparrow's Tail*
- *Diagonal Flying*
- *Ward Off*
- *Rollback, Press, Push*
- *Single Whip/Cleanse/Close Tai Chi*

These postures are performed as a slow, continuous sequence with an emphasis on relaxation, correct posture, and balance. Eventually, the practitioner may speed up the Tai Chi form, gradually, while keeping the postures correct, to the point where the movement is able to generate or emit power, as if you were involved in combat. We are now focusing on the beginning stage of practice, moving slowly, with an emphasis on the healing benefits of Tai Chi. This leads to increased awareness and vitality, and helps you to eliminate tension, regain your health, and experience the natural energy within your body and surrounding you.

The entire body should always move as one connected unit. While doing the postures, be sure that your arms are moving in conjunction with your torso: they are pushed by the legs. Your arms should not move unless the rest of your body is in motion. Remember to always line up the toes in the direction of the knees, and do not extend the knees past the toes.

As you exhale, the energy goes out through the Four Gates, the center of your palms and the center of the soles of your feet. Keep your hands in the Tai Chi hand form, relaxed, and slightly cupped, with the middle fingers downward slightly, and the pinky fingers extended. The concept is that by holding this hand form, you cause some of the energy to stagnate slightly inside the palms, making the energy there stronger. Do not move the arms from the shoulder joints only, but through the bending and releasing of the spine and chest bows.

MOUNTAIN STANCE

Stand with both feet together, palms touching two inches below your navel. Breathe deeply and close your eyes until you are calm and centered. When standing still, remember the big mountains and when moving, flow like the great rivers. On your next inhalation, open your eyes and move your arms beside your body. You are still a mountain. You have awakened, yet you are relaxed. Your brain waves are between awake and asleep, and you can sense the earth beneath you and the heavens above. You are a part of the universe.

Hands are beside the body, the middle finger touching the middle of the outer thigh. Try to sense a high spirit; a connection to the earth and heavens. Align the spine, drop the shoulders, and use deep Center of Gravity breathing. This stance can also be trained without removing your hands from your belly (two inches below the navel), to reinforce the sensation of the Lower Energy Center. You are a great mountain. You should be calm, quiet, and centered.

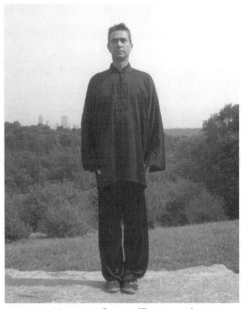

Mountain Stance (Eyes closed)

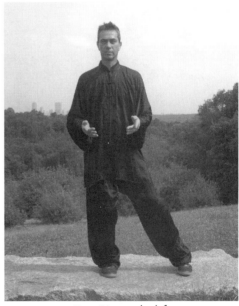

Mountain Stance (Eyes open)

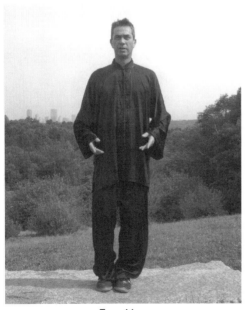

Transition

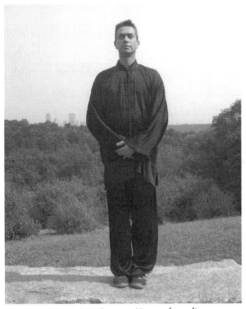

Transition to the left

BEGIN TAI CHI

Stand in Mountain stance until you are calm and centered, breathing deeply. Lift the arms slightly and hold them so that the palms face the floor, about two inches below your waist. To start, inhale and begin to raise your arms in front of your body, palms facing each other. Using the spine and chest bows, lift the arms up until the hands are at shoulder height. Be careful not to raise the shoulders or make them tight. Turn the palms downward, as if you were sliding your hands over two balls, begin exhaling, and start to lower the arms back down. Once the arms reach the solar plexus, sink the legs into Horse stance, and continue to bring the palms down, releasing the bows, and pushing your palms down as you sink.

The martial art application of this posture is for when you are facing an opponent who has their hands on top of yours, or is grabbing your wrists. You raise your arms and coil your hands around and over the outside of your opponent's hands or arms, and then push them downward, gaining the advantageous position.

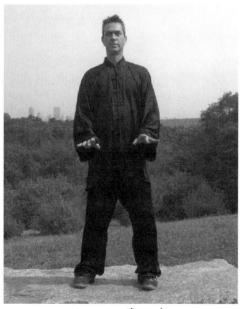

Begin Tai Chi High

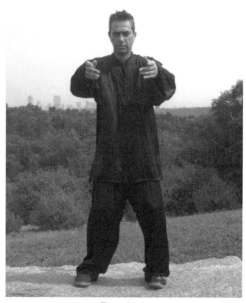

Transition

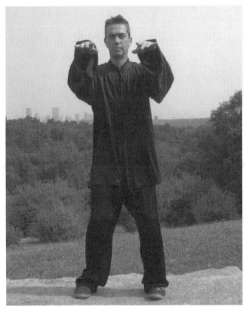

Transition

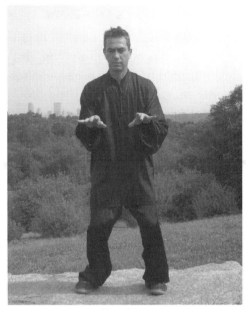

Transition

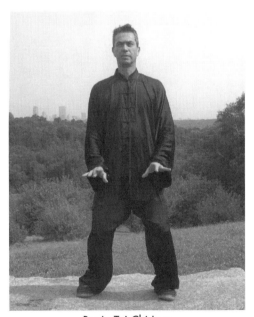

Begin Tai Chi Low

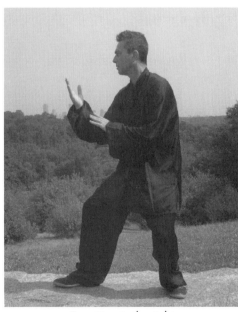

Transition to the right

GRASP THE SPARROW'S TAIL—RIGHT

Continuing from the end of Begin Tai Chi, the rest of the Tai Chi form will stay at the same height as you were in Horse stance. Your head should not move up and down throughout the various postures.

As you start to inhale, drop the right elbow, and begin to raise the right hand with the palm turned up. Simultaneously, step to the right with the right foot, pushing from the back leg. Turn toward the right into Forward stance, with the right arm raised. The left hand follows the right hand, and then touches the inside of the right wrist, supporting the action of the right arm. Exhale, step with the left leg, bringing the left foot next to the right, and place it lightly on the ground, with no weight on the left leg. At the same time, continue to extend your arms in front of you, until the right hand is at eyebrow height, with the elbows down, fingers pointing up.

The application of this posture is for intercepting an opponent's strike from the right, redirecting it upward, and opening him up for your counterattack. The left leg is "empty" to allow you to kick.

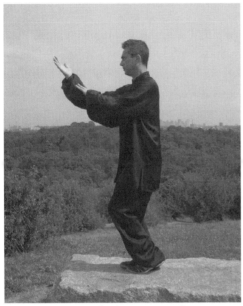

Grasp the Sparrow's Tail
on the right leg

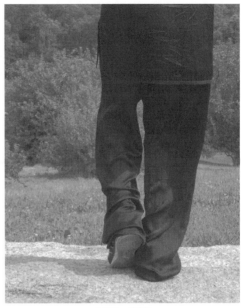

10% – 90%

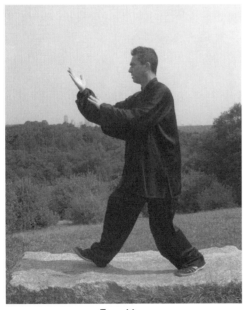

Transition

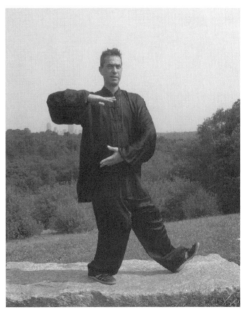

Transition to the left

DIAGONAL FLYING

Continuing from Grasp the Sparrow's Tail to Diagonal Flying is very similar. Instead of moving forward, it moves sideways. Step back with your left leg and begin to exhale. Turn on the heels into Horse stance while turning your right palm in, brushing by your face. Your right palm turns down and left palm faces up. At this point in this posture, the hands will be in front of the body, facing one another.

Pay attention to the feeling between the palms. As your left arm continues to the left, face your left palm as if it were a mirror. Continue exhaling and turn your body to your left, while changing your stance into Forward stance, left foot at a 45 degree angle, hips facing forward. Push from the back leg. As your arms move apart, imagine that you are ripping something apart with your hands. Swing your left arm to the front and the right hand to the side, with the left palm facing in and the right palm facing down. Complete your exhalation.

The application for this posture is similar to Grasp the Sparrow's Tail; it can be defensive or used as an attack.

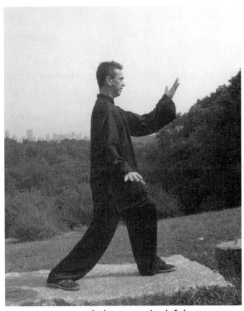

Diagonal Flying on the left leg

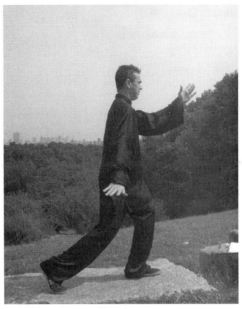

Transition

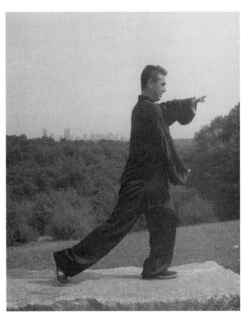

Transition

Ward Off (Peng)

Ward Off is a posture that embodies a fundamental aspect of Tai Chi practice: Ward Off energy, which is known as *Peng* (pronounced pong) in traditional Tai Chi Chuan. Ward Off energy means that your body will repel incoming force, as though you were a ball. The chest is caved inward slightly, the upper back is rounded, and the arms are expanded, with the arm joints aligned in such a way that you have a rounded feeling. This Ward Off energy is present in many other Tai Chi postures.

Continuing from Diagonal Flying, inhale and turn the body slightly to your left and rotate your left palm until it is facing downward. While bringing the right foot beside the left, cave in your chest, arc your back, and tuck in your tailbone, until you sense as if you had a ball in front of you between the palms. Do not put any weight down into the right foot; leave it "empty."

Continue inhaling, and swing the right hand to the front of the body, turning the right palm up to face the left palm. Step back with the right leg, still facing forward. Then, turn on the heels while shifting into Forward stance while swinging the right arm to your right with the arm parallel to the ground. Do not lose the sensation of the ball between your arms. As you shift forward, drop your left elbow, exhale, and push from the back leg. Forward stance ends with the hipbones facing forward. Push into the outer edge of the feet. The right palm faces in, and your left palm is under the right forearm, facing forward and slightly down. You may sense that your right arm is hugging someone, and the left palm is on his or her belly.

There are several applications for the Ward Off posture. In the first part, as you are facing the arms toward one another with a rounded feeling, you can be repelling an opponent's attack and trapping his arm. When your legs are close to one another, your groin is protected. When the right leg is "empty," it is ready to kick. When you shift to forward stance, you may trap an opponent's arm between your left palm and right forearm. Whenever you use Ward Off energy, you should feel like a ball bouncing something forward and upward.

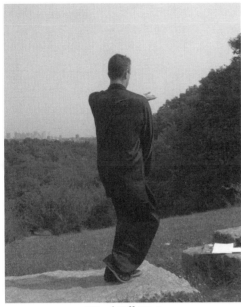

Ward Off (Yin)

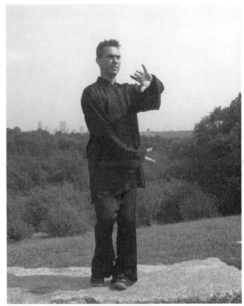

Ward Off (Yin)

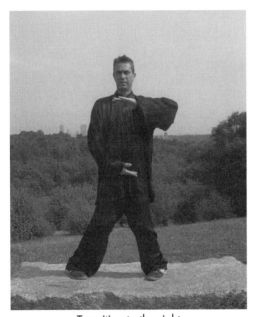

Transition to the right

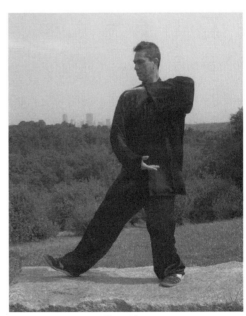

Transition

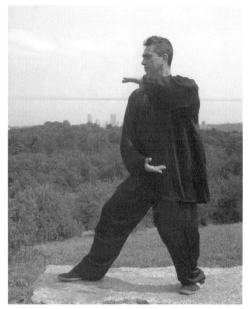

Transition

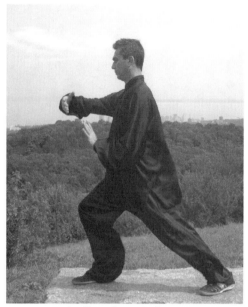

Ward Off on the right foot (Yang)
70% – 30%

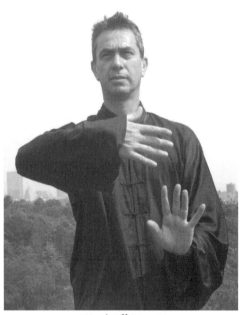

Ward Off (Yang)

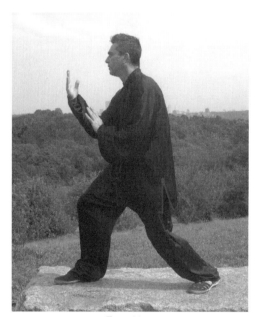

Transition

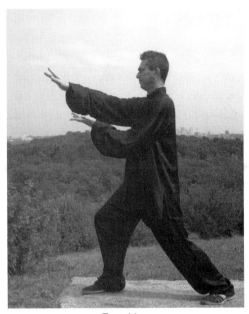

Transition

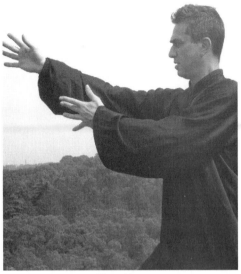

Transition

ROLLBACK, PRESS, & PUSH

Rollback (Lu)

Continuing your exhalation from Ward Off, extend you right hand upward and drop the right elbow, stretching the bows. Start to spiral the right arm forward and clockwise around an imaginary object, with the movement initiated by slightly turning the waist to the right. The right arm extends as in Grasp the Sparrow's Tail, releasing the bows, and continues the spiral movement until the right palm is facing down, while your left palm turns up.

Start inhaling, and sit back into Back stance, pulling an imaginary object between your hands back with you. Your left hand pulls back to your waist, while the right hand pulls back in front of your chest, with the right arm still extended. At the end of Rollback, the left hand makes a small circle at your waist. This is a signature movement of Yang style Tai Chi.

The application for Rollback is that you are coiling your arm around your opponent's arm and sitting back into Back stance, pulling him forward and down to expose his body for attack or to pull him entirely off balance. Your left hand holds the wrist and your right hand is on his shoulder. Rollback is usually used with a step backward.

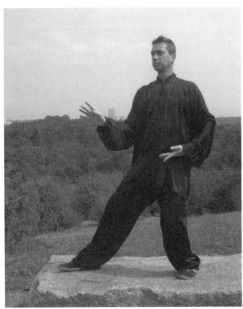

Rollback on the left leg
40% – 60%

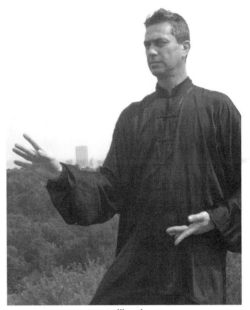

Rollback

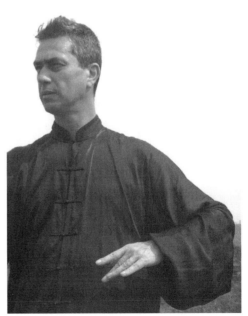

Transition

Press (Ji)

Continuing from Rollback, begin to exhale and to shift forward into Forward stance. The right arm is raised in front of the body, parallel to the ground. Here is another opportunity to feel Ward Off energy, with a rounded feeling between the right arm and the chest. Finish exhaling as the left hand moves forward to press the inside of the right wrist, and both hands press forward. Hide the fingers of the left hand behind the inside of your right wrist, so your imaginary opponent cannot grab them.

The application for this posture is that you are either pressing into an opponent quickly with both hands as a strike, or the opponent is between your hands, and you are squeezing him.

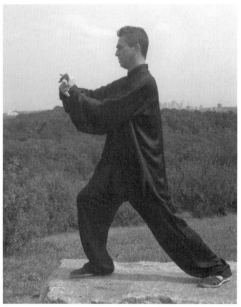

Press on the right foot
70% – 30%

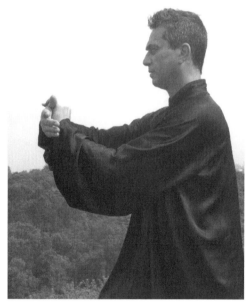

Press

Push (An)

Continuing from Press, shift your weight to the back leg, keeping you hip bones square forward. At the same time, slide your left palm over the right and separate your hands shoulder width apart in a circular, wavelike motion. Try to imitate the spirit of a mighty wave breaking on the beach (Push–Yin).

Begin to exhale as you shift your weight into Forward stance. The fingers point forward until you reach the imaginary object you will push. Then, settle your wrists downward, point the fingers up, and push forward as you finish exhaling. Make sure your head is suspended, your shoulders are relaxed and your elbows are sunk. Try to imitate the spirit of a powerful wave lifting a boat in the middle of the ocean (Push–Yang).

This Push can be applied as either a defense or an offense. You may push an opponent's attack downward to redirect the attack or to "seal" his limbs so he cannot lift them or draw them back. You may also push or strike the opponent with both hands, which requires you to have a strong feeling of being rooted to the ground, pushing from the back leg.

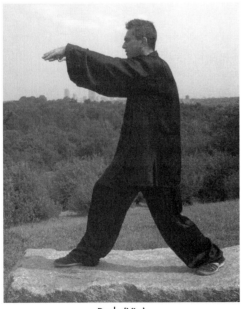

Push (Yin)
40% – 60%

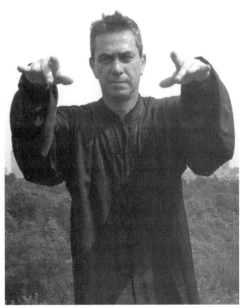

Push (Yin)

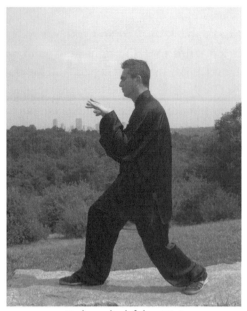

Push on the left leg (Yin)
40% – 60%

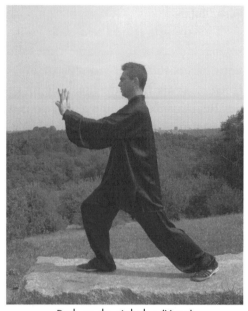

Push on the right leg (Yang)
70% – 30%

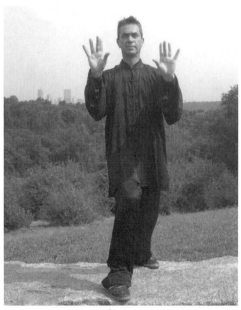

Push (Yang)

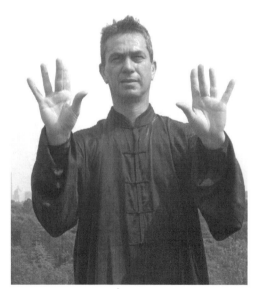

Push (Yang)

Keypoints

I first teach students to separate and break this complex sequence of Rollback, Press, Push into nine keypoints to make it easier to learn and to refine. Afterward, you emphasize these keypoints as you move through Rollback, Press, Push with continuous, smooth movement.

- One, drop the elbow.
- Two, reach up with both hands.
- Three, flip both palms.
- Four, sit back as if you are pulling a rope.
- Five, scoop or small circle with the left hand.
- Six, meet the right hand and press.
- Seven, left over right.
- Eight, sit back.
- Nine, push forward.

Rollback, Press, and Push are also fundamental energy patterns in Tai Chi, like Ward Off, and they can found within other postures throughout longer Tai Chi forms.

SINGLE WHIP

Continuing from Push, inhale and move the waist slightly to the right, allowing the upper body and then the arms to follow the whipping motion generated by your waist, so that both arms end up on the right. Continue inhaling and turn the waist to the left, while moving the feet into Horse stance. Again, let the upper body follow, so that the arms are in front of the body with the palms pointing to the right. When you reach all the way to the left, turn the waist to right, and again let the arms follow the movement. The hands will then point to the left, as they follow the arms, which are in turn pulled by the movement of the waist to the right. The movement should look like you are waving your hands together slowly underwater.

The application for Single Whip is redirection of an incoming attack away from your body. Your hands should maintain the same distance apart as if one hand is directing a wrist, and the other is directing the elbow of the same arm. For the Sunrise Tai Chi form, this is as far into the Single Whip posture that we study. Single Whip has a second part, which we will not go into here, but which you may research and train separately for longer Tai Chi forms.

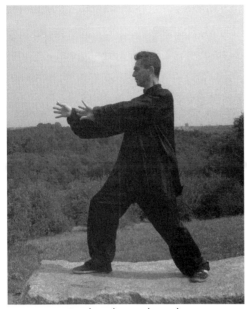

Single Whip to the right

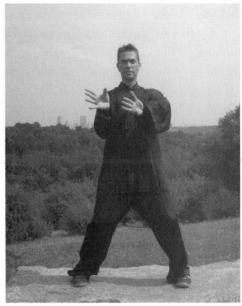

Single Whip while turning

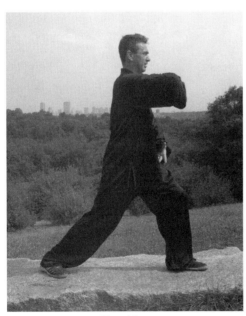

Transition

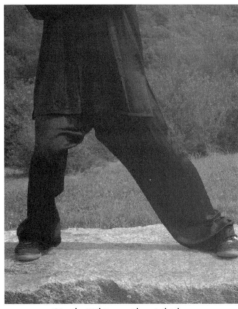

Single Whip on the right leg

CLEANSE & CLOSE TAI CHI

Once your hands are directly in front of you at the end of Single Whip, circle them both down and cross them in front of your body. Begin to inhale and continue the circle, as your arms cross up in front of your body and past your face. Then turn the palms outward, finishing the circle by dropping the hands down by your sides, and placing them on your belly over your Lower Energy Center. During Cleanse, you are gathering any impurities in your body, drawing them up through the body, and expelling them outward, far away from you, through the hands. Then, when you return your hands to your center, you are leading the clean energy in your body back to your Center of Gravity.

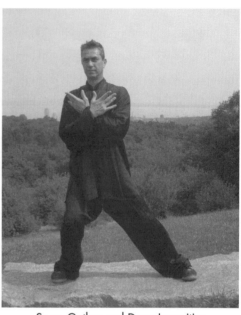

Scan, Gather and Draw Impurities

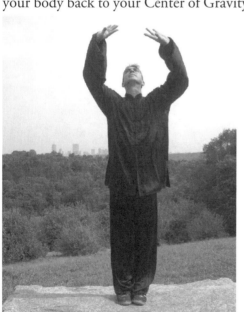

Lead and Deposit Impurities in the Stars

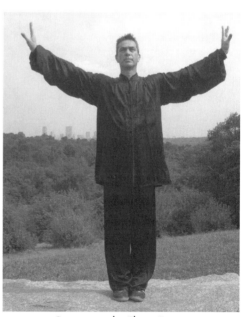

Connect to the Three Forces

Repeat the entire form again to the left, with opposite limbs.

After the second cleanse, return the palms to the front of the body, placing them over the Lower Energy Center and keeping them there for a few minutes, or as long as you like. Stand in Mountain stance and allow the energy created to return to your Lower Energy Center. This is how we Close Tai Chi.

You may also continually practice the Sunrise Tai Chi form to the right and left as many times as you like. The key to programming these movements into your body's memory, or reflexes, which are stored in the spine, is through repetition: practice, practice, practice. Always end with Close Tai Chi with the mind in the Lower Energy Center. This allows the

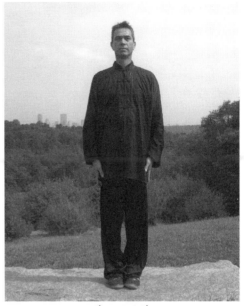

Close Tai Chi

energy you have been circulating to return to your center which calms the mind and raises the spirit.

We will focus entirely on the fundamental energy patterns taught within the Sunrise Tai Chi form, and delve more deeply into the application of each, in my next book and DVD, *Tai Chi Energy Patterns*. The concepts and theory behind these energy patterns, Ward Off, Rollback, Press, and Push (*Peng, Lu, Ji, An*) can become complex, and I have developed many exercises to train a stronger understanding of them, which are extensive and more challenging for students interested in progressing further into intermediate and advanced study of Tai Chi, including some two-person partner exercises.

End of the Sunrise Tai Chi form to the right.

The Sunrise Tai Chi form to the left.

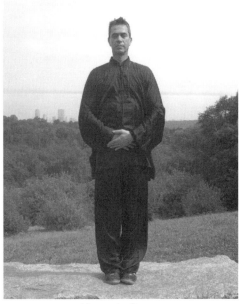

Mountain Stance

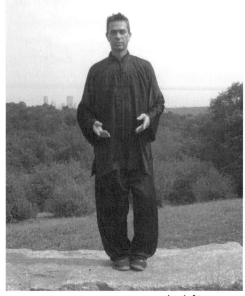

Transition to Begin Tai Chi (left)

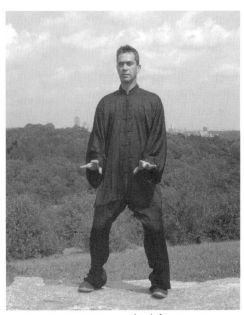

Begin Tai Chi (left)

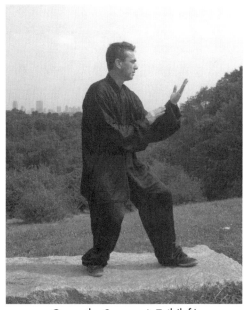

Grasp the Sparrow's Tail (left)

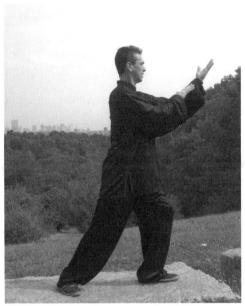

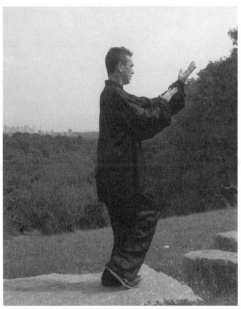

Grasp the Sparrow's Tail (left)   Grasp the Sparrow's Tail (left)

**Continue the Sunrise Tai Chi form to the left until
No Shadow, No Shape, No Form.**

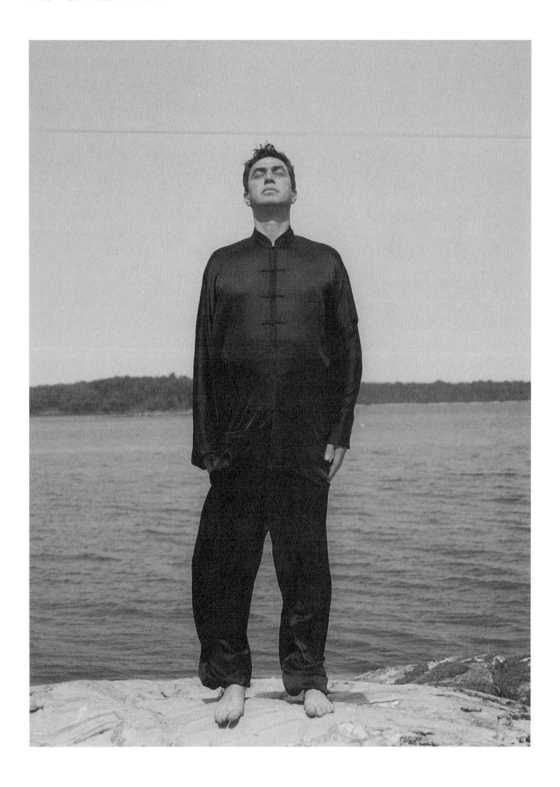

CHAPTER 6
Epilogue

During my twenty years of training full-time with world-renowned Chinese masters and leading Yoga teachers has rewarded me with gold medals in the solo Tai Chi form and Tai Chi sword, as well as in fighting competitions in North America, and Europe, in China, as well. Being exposed to such a high level of knowledge and training for six to eight hours a day, taught me that in order to have success one needs to not only emphasize the connection of the body, mind, and spirit, but to also utilize the forces around us. I have used the principles and techniques from the various Eastern arts to help individual cancer patients survive, to help the elderly cope with "unnecessary aging," and to develop and tailor a mind/body approach for the medical community to battle debilitating diseases such as cancer and arthritis. I have helped many individuals to improve their skills and reach their goals, both physical and mental. These techniques can be used by anyone interested in having a better quality of life right now.

This program is unique in that the form is trained to both the left and right, which I believe has many benefits. Also, remember that any of the exercises in this program can be done while sitting, even by those in a hospital bed, and I encourage all practitioners to experience the training while isolating the upper body. Unlike many Tai Chi publications, the main focus of this program is the internal aspects of the movements, the breathing techniques and internal visualizations, and especially the skill of tapping into earth and heaven energies. These ancient internal practices are nearly a lost art, and it is important that we pass them on to future generations.

What does it takes to get the most out of Sunrise Tai Chi program, for both martial training and for the improvement of daily performance and general health? The first step is a commitment on various levels.

Once committed, you must understand the theory behind this approach, and then learn the exercises, or mind/body prescriptions, and begin to fine tune and balance all five aspects/building blocks of our being: Body, Mind, Breath, Energy, and Spirit. You must then harmonize yourself with the three forces of earth, heaven, and human, which is a life-long journey of self-discovery and self-mastery. The *Sunrise Tai Chi* book and DVD will give you the needed fundamental first steps in this journey into the self. The basic steps are the pillars of your success. Train it until you become it.

Once you understand and train the program for a while, you will increasingly experience many benefits. You will build your muscle mass and bone density. You will free your skeleton from being a prisoner of your soft tissue. You will know how to use 80 percent effort, allowing the body to develop efficiently. You will find balance between strength and flexibility. You will increase your lung capacity and your oxygen intake, which will lead to an upgraded performance of every cell in your body. By improving your breathing, you will then be able to utilize your breathing in your visualizations and meditation.

Remember, the breath is a "banana," a tool to "Seize the Monkey Mind," calm your emotions, and to strengthen your Horse Mind, or your wisdom. When the wisdom mind is strengthened, you will be able to stay longer in a meditative state, between awake and asleep. The benefits of this have been documented for centuries in the East, and since the 1970s in the West, thanks to Herb Benson's groundbreaking work, *The Relaxation Response*. Staying longer in this meditative state will encourage production of ideal levels of healthy endorphins, neurotransmitters, and hormones, and will give your immune system an immediate boost. Your energetic circulatory system will open up, removing blockages and stagnations, improving the function of your internal organs, and your level of energy will increase tremendously. You will have a deeper understanding of the universe, and of the subtle energies around us. You will have a stronger sense of your self, the earth beneath you, and heavens above. Living with an awareness of the five building blocks and these three forces will help you live in the present moment, which is the key to being a true martial artist, and the secret that leads to improved health and longevity.

The *Sunrise Tai Chi* program is a journey in which you strike a balance between external and internal work, developing the body and mind, while tapping into sources of abundant universal energy, such as the sun. In doing so, you will be on the right path to developing a powerful fighting spirit, and a better quality of life, with countless benefits for yourself and those around you.

Glossary of Chinese Terms

How to use this glossary. This glossary will serve to help you understand Chinese words and concepts that you will encounter in this book. It also offers words that you may encounter in your continued study of Tai Chi Chuan (Taijiquan). Some included terms are not commonly known words in the Chinese language, as they exist only in Tai Chi society, such as *Peng*, which means "ward off."

Common *Qi* cavities are included, with their corresponding acupuncture cavity names, such as *Baihui* (Gv-20), which means "Hundred Meetings."

This book uses a mixture of both the Wade-Giles and Pinyin methods of transliterating Chinese to English. Usage is based on the mainstream popularity of each term, but the authors also aim to educate the reader by offering both Wade-Giles and Pinyin for many terms. Most terms in this glossary are presented only in Pinyin. Similarly, Chinese names are written in the traditional way of last name first, unless the person is more commonly known by their Westernized name, such as Lao Tzu.

An   Means "pressing or stamping." One of the eight basic moving or *Jin* patterns of *Taijiquan*. These eight moving patterns are called *Ba Men*, which means "eight doors." When *An* is done, first relax the wrist and when the hand has reached the opponent's body, immediately settle down the wrist. This action is called *Zuo Wan* in *Taijiquan* practice.

Ba Men Wu Bu   Means "eight doors and five steppings." The art of *Taijiquan* is built from eight basic moving or *Jin* patterns and five basic steppings. The eight basic moving or *Jin* patterns that can be used to handle the eight directions are called the "eight doors" (*Ba Men*) and the five stepping actions are called the "five steppings" (*Wu Bu*).

Bagua (Ba Kua)   Literally, "Eight Divinations." Also called the Eight Trigrams. In Chinese philosophy, the eight basic variations; shown in the *Yi Jing (Book of Changes)* as groups of single and broken lines.

Baihui (Gv-20)   Hundred Meetings. Name of an acupuncture cavity, which belongs to the Governing Vessel. *Baihui* is located on the crown of the head.

Can Si Jin Chan Shou Lian Xi   Silk reeling *Jin* coiling training. One of the important basic trainings in *Taijiquan*.

Chang Chuan (Changquan)   Means "long range fist or long sequence." *Chang Chuan* includes all northern Chinese long-range martial styles. *Taijiquan* is also called *Chang Chuan* simply because its sequence is long.

Cheng, Gin-Gsao (1911-1976 A.D.)   Ramel Rones' White Crane grandmaster.

Chi (Qi)   The energy pervading the universe, including the energy circulating in the human body.

Chi Kung (Qigong)   The *Gongfu* of *Qi*, which means the study of *Qi*.

Chin Na (Qin Na)   Literally means "seize control." A component of Chinese martial arts that emphasizes grabbing techniques to control your opponent's joints, in conjunction with attacking certain acupuncture cavities.

Chong Mai   Thrusting Vessel. One of the eight extraordinary vessels.

Da Lu   Large Rollback. One of the common *Taiji* techniques.

Da Mo   Bodhidharma. The 28th patriarch of Buddhism, commonly credited for popularizing the practice of Chan (Zen) Buddhism in China in 550 A.D. He settled at Shaolin temple to teach Buddhism, and developed *Qigong* exercises during his time there, greatly influencing all Chinese martial arts.

Da Qiao   To build a bridge. Refers to the *Qigong* practice of touching the roof of the mouth with the tip of the tongue to form a bridge or link between the Governing and Conception Vessels.

Da Zhou Tian   Literally, "Grand Cycle Heaven." Usually translated as "Grand Circulation." After a *Nei Dan Qigong* practitioner completes Small Circulation, he circulates his *Qi* through the entire body or exchange the *Qi* with nature.

Dai Mai   Girdle (or Belt) Vessel. One of the eight extraordinary vessels.

Dan Tian   Literally: Field of Elixir. Locations in the body that are able to store and generate *Qi* (elixir) in the body. The Upper, Middle, and Lower *Dan Tians* are located respectively between the eyebrows, at the solar plexus, and a few inches below the navel.

Dao   The "way," by implication the "natural way."

Dao De Jing (Tao Te Ching)   *Morality Classic*. Written by Lao Zi during the Zhou Dynasty (1122-934 B.C.).

Dazhui (Gv-14)   Big Vertebra. Name of an acupuncture cavity that belongs to the Governing Vessel.

Deng Shan Bu   Climbing Mountain Stance, or Forward Stance. One of the basic fundamental stances in northern martial arts. Also called Bow and Arrow Stance (*Gong Jian Bu*).

Dian Xue   *Dian* means "to point and exert pressure" and *Xue* means "the cavities." *Dian Xue* refers to those *Qin Na* techniques that specialize in attacking acupuncture cavities to immobilize or kill an opponent.

Dong Jin   Understanding *Jin*. One of the *Jins* that uses the feeling of the skin to sense the opponent's energy.

Du Mai   Usually translated "Governing Vessel." One of the eight *Qi* vessels.

Fan Hu Xi (Ni Hu Xi)   Reverse Breathing. Also commonly called Daoist Breathing.

Fan Tong Hu Xi   Back to childhood breathing. A breathing training in *Nei Dan Qigong* through which the practitioner tries to regain control of the muscles in the lower abdomen. Also called "abdominal breathing (*Fu Shi Hu Xi*)."

Fu Sui Xi   Skin and Marrow Breathing. Skin breathing is considered as *Yang* while marrow breathing is classified as *Yin*.

Fu Xi   Skin Breathing. One of the *Nei Dan Qigong* breathing techniques in which the *Qi* is led to the skin surface.

Ha   A *Yang* sound that is used to manifest martial power to its highest efficiency.

Han Xiong Ba Bei   Means to contain or draw in the chest and arc the back.

Han, Ching-Tang   A well-known Chinese martial artist, especially in Taiwan. Master Han is Ramel Rones' Long Fist *kung fu* great grandmaster.

Hen   A *Yin Qigong* sound that is the opposite of the *Yang Ha* sound. This sound is commonly used to lead the *Qi* inward and to store it in the bone marrow. This sound can also be used for an attack when the manifestation of only partial power is desired.

Hou Tian Qi   Post-birth *Qi* or post-heaven *Qi*. This *Qi* is converted from the Essence of food and air and is classified as "fire *Qi*" since it can make your body too *Yang*.

Hua   To neutralize.

Huan Jing Bu Nao   Literally, to return the Essence to nourish the brain. A Daoist *Qigong* training process wherein *Qi* that has been converted from Essence is lead to the brain to nourish it.

Huang Ting   Yellow Yard. 1. A yard or hall in which Daoists, who often wore yellow robes, meditate together. 2. In Daoist *Qigong*, the place in the center of the body where Fire *Qi* and Water *Qi* are mixed to generate a spiritual embryo.

Huiyin   Perineum. An acupuncture cavity belonging to the Conception Vessel.

Hun   The soul. Commonly used with the word *Ling*, which means spirit. Daoists believe that a human being's *Hun* and *Po* originate with his Original *Qi (Yuan Qi),* and separate from the physical body at death.

Huo Lu   Fire path. One of the paths in Small Circulation meditation.

Ji   Means "to squeeze" or "to press."

Ji Gong   Spine Bow. The bow formed from the spine, which is able to store the *Jin.*

Jia Dan Tian   False *Dan Tian*. It is called *Qihai* (Co-6) in acupuncture. This place, the front of the belly, is able to produce *Qi*. However, it cannot store *Qi* efficiently.

Jiaji   Squeeze the Spine. The Daoist name of a spot on the spine in Small Circulation meditation practice. This spot is called *Lingtai* (Gv-10) (i.e., spirit's platform) in acupuncture.

Jin, Shao-Feng   Ramel Rones' White Crane kung fu great grandmaster.

Jing (Jin)   Chinese martial power. A combination of *Li* (muscular power) and *Qi*.

Jing Qi   Essence *Qi*. The *Qi* which has been converted from Original Essence.

Jing-Shen   Essence-Spirit. Often translated as the "Spirit of Vitality." Raised spirit (raised by the *Qi* that is converted from Essence) which is restrained by the *Yi*.

Kao   Means "to lean or to press against." In *Taijiquan*, it means to bump someone off balance.

Kao, Tao   Dr. Yang, Jwing-Ming's first *Taijiquan* master.

Kua   The area on the external hip joint is called "external *Kua*" (*Wai Kua*) whereas the area on the inner side of the hip joints (i.e., groin area) is called "internal *Kua*" (*Nei Kua*).

Kung (Gong)   Means "energy" or "hard work."

Kung Fu (Gongfu)   Means "energy-time." Anything which will take time and energy to learn or to accomplish is called *Kung Fu*.

Lao Zu (or Lao Zi) Considered the creator, or first compiler, of Daoism, also called *Li Er*. Author of the book, *Dao De Jing*.

Laogong (P-8) Labor's Palace. A cavity name. On the Pericardium Channel in the center of the palm.

Li The power that is generated from muscular strength.

Li, Mao-Ching Ramel Rones' Long Fist *kung fu* grandmaster.

Lian Jing Hua Qi To refine the Essence and convert it into *Qi*.

Lian Qi Hua Shen To refine the *Qi* to nourish the spirit. Leading *Qi* to the head to nourish the brain and spirit.

Lian Qi Sheng Hua To train the *Qi* and sublimate it. A *Xi Sui Jing* training process by which the *Qi* is led to the *Huang Ting* or the brain.

Liang, Shou-Yu Ramel Rones' *Xingyiquan* (*Hsing-Yi Chuan*) and *Baguazhang* (*Pa Kua Chang*) master.

Lingtai (Gv-10) Spiritual Station. In acupuncture, a cavity on the back. In *Qigong*, it refers to the Upper *Dan Tian*. In Daoist society, the *Lingtai* cavity is called *Jia Ji*.

Li Qi *Li* is muscular power, while *Qi* is inner energy. *Li-Qi* means "to manifest the inner energy into physical power," which means *Jin*.

Liu Yi The six arts—consisting of writing, music, archery, chariot driving, learning rhetoric, and mathematics—which ancient Chinese scholars were required to master.

Lu Means "to rollback."

Luo The small *Qi* channels that branch out from the primary *Qi* channels and are connected to the skin and to the bone marrow.

Mingmen (Gv-4) Life's Door. Name of an acupuncture cavity that belongs to the Governing Vessel.

Na Jin Controlling *Jins*. The *Jins* that are able to control the opponent through his joints or tendons.

Nei Shen Literally, internal kidneys. In Chinese medicine and *Qigong*, the real kidneys; while *Wai Shen* (external kidneys) refer to the testicles.

Nei Shi Literally, internal vision. It implies feeling to the inner body. It also means "internal inspection through inner feeling."

Nei Shi Gongfu   *Nei Shi* means "to look internally," so *Nei Shi Gongfu* refers to the art of looking inside yourself to read the state of your health and the condition of your *Qi*.

Ni Wan or Ni Wan Gong   Mud pill, or mud pill palace. Daoist *Qigong* terminology for an area in the brain.

Peng   Means "to ward off."

Po   Vigorous life force. The *Po* is considered to be the inferior or animal soul. It is the animal or sentient life that is an innate part of the body, which at death returns to the earth with the rest of the body. When someone is in high spirits and gets vigorously involved in some activity, it is said he has *Po Li*, which means he has "vigorous strength or power."

Qigong (Chi Kung)   The *Gongfu* of *Qi*, which means the study of *Qi*.

Ren Mai   Usually translated "Conception Vessel."

Renzhong (Gv-26)   An acupuncture cavity under the nose.

San Guan   Three gates. In Small Circulation training, the three cavities on the Governing Vessel which are usually obstructed and must be opened.

Shang Dan Tian   Upper *Dan Tian*. The brain; it is the residence of the *Shen* (spirit).

Shaolin   A Buddhist temple in Henan Province, famous for its martial arts.

Shen   Spirit. According to Chinese *Qigong*, the *Shen* resides at the Upper *Dan Tian* (the third eye).

Shen Gu   Spirit Valley. Formed by the two lobes of the brain, with the Upper *Dan Tian* at the exit.

Shen Xi   Spirit breathing. The stage of *Qigong* training where the spirit is coordinated with the breathing.

Shi San Shi   Thirteen Patterns. *Taijiquan* is also called *Shi San Shi*, since it is constructed from these thirteen moving patterns.

Shuai Jiao   Means "wrestling."

Shuang Xiu   Double cultivation. A *Qigong* training method in which *Qi* is exchanged with a partner in order to balance the *Qi* in both people.

Shuang Zhong   Means "double weighting" or "double layering." It means when the opponent has placed a weight or pressure on you, you respond by meeting that pressure with equal or greater pressure of your own. The consequence is stagnation. When this happens, mutual resistance will be generated.

Shui Lu   Water Path. One of the meditation paths in which the *Qi* is led upward through the spinal cord (Thrusting Vessel, *Chong Mai*) to nourish the brain.

Si Liang Po Qian Jin   Means to use four ounces to repel (i.e., neutralize) one thousand pounds.

Si Liu Bu   Four-Six Stance, or Back Stance. One of the basic stances in northern styles of martial arts training, with 60 percent of the weight on the rear leg.

Sun Wu   Also named Sun Zi. A famous strategist who lived around 557 B.C. He wrote the book *Sun Zi's Fighting Strategies* (*Sun Zi Bing Fa*). This book is commonly translated as *The Art of War*.

Tai Chi Chuan (Taijiquan)   Grand Ultimate Fist. A Chinese internal martial style that is based on the theory of *Taiji* (grand ultimate).

Taiji   Means "grand ultimate." It is this force that generates two poles, *Yin* and *Yang*.

Taiji Quan Chan Shou Lian Xi   *Taiji* (Tai Chi) circle sticking hands training. One of the most important trainings in Yang-style *Taijiquan* (Tai Chi Chuan). This training is used to train listening, understanding, sticking, adhering, connecting, and following. In Chen style, it is called "Silk reeling *Jin* coiling training" (*Chan Si Jin Chan Shou Lian Xi*).

Taiwan   An island to the southeast of mainland China. Also known as Formosa.

Ti Xi   Body breathing or skin breathing. In *Qigong*, the exchanging of *Qi* with the surrounding environment through the skin.

Tian Ling Gai   Literally, heaven spiritual cover. A person's head is considered to be heaven, and the crown is called "heaven spiritual cover" by Daoist society. This place is called *Baihui* (Gv-20) in acupuncture.

Tian Ren He Yi   Literally, "Heaven and man unified as one." A high level of *Qigong* practice in which a *Qigong* practitioner, through meditation, is able to communicate his *Qi* with heaven's *Qi*.

Tian Yan   Heaven Eye. The third eye or Upper *Dan Tian*.

Tiao Qi   To regulate the *Qi*.

Tiao Shen   To regulate the body.

Tiao Shen   To regulate the spirit.

Tiao Xi   To regulate the breathing.

Tiao Xin   To regulate the emotional mind.

Ting Jin   Listening *Jin*. A special training that uses the skin to feel the opponent's energy and uses this feeling to further understand his intention.

Tui Na   Means "to push and grab." A category of Chinese massages for healing and injury treatment.

Wang, Zong-Yue   A well-known Tai Chi master during the late Qing Dynasty who wrote many comprehensive Tai Chi Chuan documents. He is popularly studied by Tai Chi Chuan practitioners today.

Wei Qi   Protective *Qi* or Guardian *Qi*. The *Qi* at the surface of the body, which generates a shield to protect the body from negative external influences such as colds.

Weilu   Tailbone. A Daoist name. This cavity is called *Changqiang* (Gv-1) in acupuncture.

Wen Huo   Scholar fire. Through soft and slender breathing, the *Qi* (i.e., fire) can be built up gently at the abdominal area.

Wu Bu   Five steppings. They include: forward, backward, left, right, and center.

Wu Huo   Martial fire. Through fast and short breathing techniques, the *Qi* (i.e., fire) can be built up to an abundant level for the physical manifestation in a short time. However, through this technique, though the fire can be built up in a fast way, it is hard to keep it in the body.

Wu Xin   Five Centers or Five Gates. The face, the *Laogong* cavities in both palms, and the *Yongquan* cavities on the bottoms of both feet.

Wu Xin Xi   Five Gates Breathing.

Wu Xing   Five Phases, including: metal (*Jin*), wood (*Mu*), water (*Shui*), fire (*Huo*), and earth (*Tu*).

Wudang (Wu Tang) Mountain   Located in Hubei Province in China.

Wuji   Means "no extremity."

Wuji Hu Xi (Wuji Xi)   *Wuji* Breathing. Keeping the mind at the Real *Dan Tian* during breathing practice.

Xi Sui Jing   Literally: *Washing Brain/Marrow Classic*, usually called *Marrow/Brain Washing Classic*. Credited to Bodhidharma (Da Mo) around 550 A.D., this work discusses *Qigong* for washing the marrow or cleaning the brain by *Qi* nourishment.

Xia Dan Tian   Lower elixir field. Located in the lower abdomen, it is believed to be the residence of water *Qi* (Original *Qi*) (*Yuan Qi*). This cavity in acupuncture is called *Qihai* (Co-6) which means "*Qi* ocean."

Xian Tian Qi   Pre-Birth *Qi* or Pre-Heaven *Qi*. Also called *Dan Tian Qi*. The *Qi*, which is converted from Original Essence and is stored in the Lower *Tian*. Considered to be "water *Qi*," it is able to calm the body.

Xiao Lu   Small rollback.

Xin   Means "heart." *Xin* means "the mind generated from emotional disturbance."

Xin Yuan Yi Ma   *Xin*-monkey and *Yi*-horse. *Xin* (i.e., heart) is related to the emotional mind, is like a monkey, and is hard to keep steady and calm. *Yi* is wise and logical thinking, which is like a horse that can be calm and keep still.

Xinzhu Xian   Birthplace of Dr. Yang, Jwing-Ming in Taiwan.

Xiong Gong   Chest bow. The bow formed from the chest, which is able to store the *Jin* significantly.

Xu Ling Ding Jin   An insubstantial energy leads the head upward. A secret *Taijiquan* phrase which helps a *Taijiquan* practitioner keep the head upright and the neck relaxed.

Yang   Too sufficient. One of the two poles. The other is *Yin*.

Yang, Ban-Hou (1837-1892 A.D.)   Yang, Lu-Shan's second son. Also called Yang, Yu. A second generation practitioner of *Yang-style* Taijiquan.

Yi   Wisdom mind. The mind generated from wise judgment.

Yi Jin Jing   Literally: *Changing Muscle/Tendon Classic*, usually called *The Muscle/Tendon Changing Classic*. Credited to Bodhidharma (Da Mo) around 550 A.D., this work discusses *Wai Dan* (External Elixir) *Qigong* training for strengthening the physical body.

Yin   Deficient. One of the two poles. The other is *Yang*.

Yin Shui   *Yin* Water. The *Qi* stored at the Real *Dan Tian* is called *Yin Shui*, since keeping the *Qi* here may keep you calm.

Yongquan (K-1)   Bubbling Well or Gushing Spring. Name of an acupuncture cavity belonging to the Kidney Primary *Qi* Channel in center of sole of the feet.

Yuan Jing   Original Essence. The fundamental, original substance inherited from your parents; it is converted into Original *Qi*.

Yuan Qi   Original *Qi*. Created from the Original Essence inherited from your parents.

Zen (Chan)   A school of Mahayana Buddhism that asserts that spiritual enlightenment can be attained through meditation, self-contemplation, and intuition.

Zhang, San-Feng   A monk from Wudang commonly credited as the creator of *Taijiquan* during the Song Dynasty in China (960-1127 A.D.).

Special Thanks to Dr. Yang, Jwing-Ming for his extensive research
and knowledge which comprise the contents of this glossary.

Recommended Readings

Benson, Herbert and Miriam Z. Clipper. *The Relaxation Response*. New York: Harper Paperbacks, 2000.

Calais-Germain, Blandine. *Anatomy in Movement*. Translated by Nicole Commarmond, edited by Stephen Anderson. Seattle: Eastland Press, 1993.

Frantzis, Bruce Kumar. *Opening the Energy Gates of Your Body. Chi Gung for Lifelong Heath*. Berkeley, CA: North Atlantic, 1993.

Frantzis, Bruce Kumar. *Relaxing Into Your Being*. Berkeley, CA: North Atlantic Press, 2001.

Frantzis, Bruce Kumar. *The Great Stillness*. Fairfax, CA: Clarity Press, 1999.

Kaptchuk, Ted. *The Web That Has No Weaver: Understanding Chinese Medicine*. New York:McGraw-Hill, 2000.

Nelson, Miriam and Sarah Wernick. *Strong Women Stay Young*. NY: Bantam, 2000.

Yang, Jwing-Ming. *Qigong for Health and Martial Arts*. 2nd ed. Boston, MA: YMAA Publication Center, 1998.

Yang, Jwing-Ming. *Qigong Meditation—Embryonic Breathing*. Boston, MA: YMAA Publication Center, 2003.

Yang, Jwing-Ming. *Qigong, the Secret of Youth: Da Mo's Muscle/Tendon Changing, Marrow/Brain Washing Classics. The Secret of Youth*. Boston, MA: YMAA Publication Center, 2000.

Yang, Jwing-Ming. *Tai Chi Theory and Martial Power*. Boston, MA: YMAA Publication Center, 1996.

Yang, Jwing-Ming. *The Root of Chinese Qigong*. 2nd ed. Boston, MA: YMAA Publication Center, 1997.

www.mindandlife.org – articles and publications

Index

abdominal muscles 18, 22-24, 44
alignment 82
An 171
ankles 64-65
arthritis 90
aura energy 31-32
back muscles 22-24
Back stance 100, 112, 118
baton energy center 30-31
baton visualization 29-30
baton/bubble breathing visualization 32-34
Begin Tai Chi posture 97, 107, 158
bone marrow-skin breathing 32-34
Bow and Arrow stance 99
breath 16
Breath block 153
breath, exhalation 16-17
breath, inhalation 16
breathing
    baton/bubble 38-39
    bubble 45
    buddhist 24
    Four Gates 34-35, 54
    spiritual 36-39
    taoist 24
    Three Chambers 51
    Two Bows 55
bubble breathing 45
bubble visualization 31-32
calf muscles 57
Cat stance 101
Center of Gravity Energy Center 21-30
cervical spine 18-21
chambers 51
Chen family 5-6
chest 18-21
chin 86
Cleanse posture 176
cleansing the body 46
Crane Lifts to Heaven exercise 74
Dan Tian 21-22
Dao Yin 3-4
Diagonal Flying 128, 130, 162
double-weighting 6

down force 78
earth energy 47
Eastern arts 12-13
Elbows 88
Elixir Field 21-22
Emperor/Empress position 42, 76
Empty Moon 22-24
Empty stance 101, 110, 114
Empty/Full Moon breathing 118
energy ball 24-26
energy baton 30-31
energy gates 34-36
energy patterns 173
exhalation 6-7, 51,156
external baton visualization 28-30
feet 92
Fire Set exercise 67, 68
five building blocks 153
five elements 153
flexibility 86
forces, upward and down 17-21, 78
Forty Percent-Sixty Percent stance 100
Forward stance 99, 112, 116
four gates breathing 34-36
Full Moon 22-24
gates, energy 34-36
Governing Vessel 35-36
Graham, Martha 17-18
Grasp the Sparrow's Tail 121, 122, 125
Guardian Energy 32
Hamstring Stretch 57
hand form 156
head 84
Heavenly Gate 47
heels 92
hips 66-67
Horse Mind 16-17, 24
Horse stance 98, 108, 114
Hsu, Hsuan-P'ing 4
impurities 46
inhalation 16
insubstantial 96, 104, 116
internal visualization 14-16
Ji 170

Joints 58
knees 90
kua 114
Lao Tzu 3, 6
Look to the Left and Look to the Right exercise
    60-61
Loosening the Neck 60
lower back 52-53
Lu 168
lumbar spine 18
lung capacity 76
lungs 51
martial arts, four basic principles 4
Massage, Organ 49
meditation 12-13
meditation, sitting 42
Meditation, Standing 44
Mind and Energy blocks 154
mind/body prescriptions 14, 71
Monkey Mind 16-17, 24
Mountain Climbing stance 99, 112
Mountain stance 96, 105, 156
multi-visualizing 35-38
muscle mass 70
muscles 22-24, 71
muscles, meditation and 44
near-sleep state 12-13
neck 60-61, 84
No Thought 16-17, 35-38
Nourishing 47, 75
organ massage 49
Osteoporosis 69-70
oxygen intake 76
Peng 164
Pigeon Picks Up the Seeds 61
pituitary gland energy center 26-28, 29-30, 78
postures 155, 156
postures, eight basic 4
postures, fundamental thirteen 4
postures, sitting 15-16
Press 136, 138, 146, 152, 170
Push 140, 142, 146, 152, 171
Qi energy 3-4, 7, 14-16, 21-22, 56
Regulating without Regulating 35-38
relaxation 17-18
resistance 70-71

Rollback 146, 152, 168
sacrum 73
sarcopenia 70
shallow breathing 42
shoulders 84
Single Whip posture 144, 174
sitting meditation 42
sitting posture 15-16
Spirit block 154
spiritual breathing 36-39
Spiritual Valley 36-39, 78
squatting down 64
stances 95, 155
stances, training 96
standing exercises 24-26
standing meditation 44
stationary drills 120
steppings, five directional movements 5
strength 86
Stretch, Flamingo 61-62
stretching 41, 52-53
    ankles 64
    hamstrings 57
    knees 64
    neck 60-61
substantial 96, 104, 116
sun energy 78
Sun Nourishing exercise 75, 79
Tai Chi 1
Tai Chi Thirteen Postures 4
Tai Chi Ball 55-56
Tai Chi Chuan
    Chen family 5-6
    combat 6
    five family styles 6
    forms 1-3
    hand form 95
    history 3, 5-6
    stances 95
    Wu Style 5-6
    Yang-style 1-3, 6
taiji See Tai Chi
taijiquan See Tai Chi Chuan
Tame the Tiger stance 103, 114
Tao Te Ching 3
taoist breathing 24

temporomandibular joints 43
tension 17-18
The Way of Virtue 3
Third Eye 36-39
Thirteen Postures of Tai Chi 4
thoracic spine 18-21, 78
three spheres 18
torso 18
training 13-14
trigrams 4
Tu Na 3-4
Turtle Back 136
Two Bows Breathing 55
up and down forces 78
up force 18-21, 78
Up Like Smoke, Down Like a Feather exercises
   69
Upper Energy Center 78
visualization 45
visualization, baton 29-30
visualization, baton/bubble breathing 32-33
visualization, bubble 31-32
visualization, external baton 28-29
visualization, pituitary gland energy center 26-28
Vitamin L exercise 52
Walk and Kick Back 67
Walk Like a Warrior exercises 68
Ward Off 134, 146, 152
Ward Off posture 132, 164
warm up 41
Wei Qi 32
weight shifting 116
Wisdom Mind 16-17
Wu Style Tai Chi Chuan 5-6
Wuji 3
Wuji stance 97
Yan Wu Di 5-6
Yang style Tai Chi Chuan 6
Yang, Cheng-Fu 86
Yang, Lu-Chan 5-6
Yang, Pan-Hou 5-6
Yang-style Tai Chi Chuan 1-3
Yi 16-17
Yin-Yang 3
Zen meditation 16
Zhang, San-Feng 4

About the Authors

Ramel 'Rami' Rones has witnessed first hand the profound long-term benefits of Tai Chi and *Qigong* practice. Since 1989, he has been working to improve the lives of cancer and arthritis patients. He is a Scientific Consultant of Mind/Body Therapies at Dana Farber Cancer Institute, Harvard and Tufts Medical Schools in Boston, MA.

A prolific writer on the subjects of healing and the internal arts, he is co-author of numerous scientific publications, articles, and is working on the book *The Power of One: Awakening the Warrior Within* with Elian Littman.

He is the creator of the Tai Chi component of the "Secrets of Aging" Science Museum traveling exhibition (Boston, Columbus, Los Angeles, Fort Worth, Philadelphia, Minneapolis) 2000 to 2004.

A senior disciple of renowned teacher and author Dr. Yang, Jwing-Ming Ph.D. in Boston, MA since the 1980s, Ramel is a Gold medalist in Internal and External Martial Arts: Three-time Gold Medalist in Shanghai, China for Tai Chi, External & Internal Weapons (Grand National Championship 1994), and Gold Medalist for Tai Chi & Kung Fu Sword, 1994. From 1991 to 1993, Ramel earned gold medals for Tai Chi, Pushing Hands, and Tai Chi Sword in the International North American Chinese Martial Arts Competition.

Ramel works to improve the quality of life of his many students, improve their martial arts skills, and to help some cope with cancer, arthritis, and other serious ailments using the principles taught in this book and DVD. *Sunrise Tai Chi* is his first book.

David Silver has been a student of the ancient Chinese art of *Qigong* since the 1990s, and became certified to carry on the teaching of *Qigong* by Master Yang, Jwing-Ming in Boston, MA. He works as a producer and director of instructional health and martial arts DVDs, and teaches group and private *Qigong* classes. David has also worked as editor of Dr. Yang, Jwing-Ming's *Qigong* books, and has contributed his research/writing skills to many other published materials. *Sunrise Tai Chi* is his first book.

SUNRISE TAI CHI— DVD
Ramel Rones

Captured in high-definition in the beautiful Boston Arboretum, this simplified, short Tai Chi sequence is practiced to both the left and right for balance. Sunrise Tai Chi was created as a comprehensive introduction to authentic Tai Chi, which will allow you to fine-tune your practice before moving on to more complex Tai Chi. It includes suggestions for intermediate and advanced students, to help you grow and improve over time.

- Revitalize your health and well being through deep relaxation, breath, meditation, stretching and strengthening techniques.
- Apply core principles of Tai Chi, Qigong, and Yoga together with Mind/Body Science to tap into the abundant universal energy.
- Prevent injuries and boost your immune system to heal chronic conditions, including Arthritis, Osteoporosis, Sarcopenia, and Cancer.

Complements the book *Sunrise Tai Chi.*

220 min. • DVD9-NTSC • ISBN-10: 1-59439-027-4 •
ISBN-13: 978-1-59439-027-2

  SKILL LEVEL Ⅰ Ⅱ Ⅲ

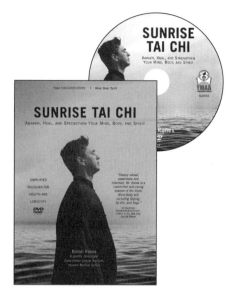

Companion DVD!

TAI CHI ENERGY PATTERNS—DVD
Taijiquan Solo & Partner Exercises
Ramel Rones

Captured in High-Definition in the beautiful Harvard Arboretum, this 2-DVD Set offers unparalleled quality and extensive navigation. Detailed computer animations of the energy circulating in the body make the once-secret skills of internal cultivation easier to understand and learn.

Ramel Rones instructs essential movements and training exercises, with a focus on four popular Tai Chi Patterns: Ward Off, Rollback, Press, and Push (Peng, Lu, Ji, An). You will learn to develop and utilize the internal (Qi) energy that can be found within all Tai Chi movements. The energy circulation, mental visualizations, extensive breathing techniques, and physical skills taught in this program can be applied to all Tai Chi styles.

You may study the instructional segment in a formal classroom setting, or follow along as each movement is demonstrated. This advanced DVD also offers viewing choices of a 30-Minute Workout, Sitting Workout, or a Partner Workout.

2DVD Set • 385 minutes • ISBN: 1-59439-052-5 •
ISBN-13: 978-1-59439-052-4

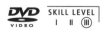 SKILL LEVEL Ⅰ Ⅱ Ⅲ

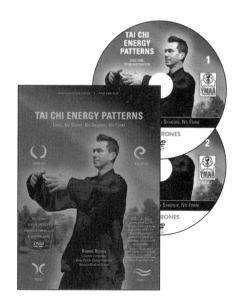

BOOKS FROM YMAA

6 HEALING MOVEMENTS	B906
101 REFLECTIONS ON TAI CHI CHUAN	B868
108 INSIGHTS INTO TAI CHI CHUAN — A STRING OF PEARLS	B582
A WOMAN'S QIGONG GUIDE	B833
ADVANCING IN TAE KWON DO	B072X
ANCIENT CHINESE WEAPONS	B671
ANALYSIS OF SHAOLIN CHIN NA 2ND ED.	B0002
ARTHRITIS RELIEF — CHINESE QIGONG FOR HEALING & PREVENTION, 3RD ED.	B0339
BACK PAIN RELIEF — CHINESE QIGONG FOR HEALING & PREVENTION 2ND ED.	B0258
BAGUAZHANG	B300
CHIN NA IN GROUND FIGHTING	B663
CHINESE FAST WRESTLING — THE ART OF SAN SHOU KUAI JIAO	B493
CHINESE FITNESS — A MIND / BODY APPROACH	B37X
CHINESE TUI NA MASSAGE	B043
COMPLETE CARDIOKICKBOXING	B809
COMPREHENSIVE APPLICATIONS OF SHAOLIN CHIN NA	B36X
DR. WU'S HEAD MASSAGE—ANTI-AGING AND HOLISTIC HEALING THERAPY	B0576
EIGHT SIMPLE QIGONG EXERCISES FOR HEALTH, 2ND ED.	B523
ESSENCE OF SHAOLIN WHITE CRANE	B353
ESSENCE OF TAIJI QIGONG, 2ND ED.	B639
EXPLORING TAI CHI	B424
FIGHTING ARTS	B213
INSIDE TAI CHI	B108
KATA AND THE TRANSMISSION OF KNOWLEDGE	B0266
LIUHEBAFA FIVE CHARACTER SECRETS	B728
MARTIAL ARTS ATHLETE	B655
MARTIAL ARTS INSTRUCTION	B024X
MARTIAL WAY AND ITS VIRTUES	B698
MIND/BODY FITNESS	B876
NATURAL HEALING WITH QIGONG — THERAPEUTIC QIGONG	B0010
NORTHERN SHAOLIN SWORD, 2ND ED.	B85X
OKINAWA'S COMPLETE KARATE SYSTEM — ISSHIN RYU	B914
POWER BODY	B760
PRINCIPLES OF TRADITIONAL CHINESE MEDICINE	B99X
QIGONG FOR HEALTH & MARTIAL ARTS 2ND ED.	B574
QIGONG FOR LIVING	B116
QIGONG FOR TREATING COMMON AILMENTS	B701
QIGONG MASSAGE 2ND ED. —FUND. TECHNIQUES FOR HEALTH AND RELAXATION	B0487
QIGONG MEDITATION — EMBRYONIC BREATHING	B736
QIGONG MEDITATION—SMALL CIRCULATION	B0673
QIGONG, THE SECRET OF YOUTH	B841
ROOT OF CHINESE QIGONG, 2ND ED.	B507
SHIHAN TE — THE BUNKAI OF KATA	B884
SUNRISE TAI CHI	B0838
SURVIVING ARMED ASSAULTS	B0711
TAEKWONDO — ANCIENT WISDOM FOR THE MODERN WARRIOR	B930
TAEKWONDO — SPIRIT AND PRACTICE	B221
TAO OF BIOENERGETICS	B289
TAI CHI BOOK	B647
TAI CHI CHUAN — 24 & 48 POSTURES	B337
TAI CHI CHUAN MARTIAL APPLICATIONS, 2ND ED.	B442
TAI CHI CONNECTIONS	B0320
TAI CHI SECRETS OF THE ANCIENT MASTERS	B71X
TAI CHI SECRETS OF THE WÜ & LI STYLES	B981
TAI CHI SECRETS OF THE WU STYLE	B175
TAI CHI SECRETS OF THE YANG STYLE	B094
TAI CHI THEORY & MARTIAL POWER, 2ND ED.	B434
TAI CHI WALKING	B23X
TAIJI CHIN NA	B378
TAIJI SWORD, CLASSICAL YANG STYLE	B744
TAIJIQUAN, CLASSICAL YANG STYLE	B68X
TAIJIQUAN THEORY OF DR. YANG, JWING-MING	B432
THE CUTTING SEASON	B0821
THE WAY OF KATA—A COMPREHENSIVE GUIDE TO DECIPHERING MARTIAL APPS.	B0584
THE WAY OF KENDO AND KENJITSU	B0029
THE WAY OF SANCHIN KATA	B0845
TRADITIONAL CHINESE HEALTH SECRETS	B892
TRADITIONAL TAEKWONDO—CORE TECHNIQUES, HISTORY, AND PHILOSOPHY	B0665
XINGYIQUAN, 2ND ED.	B416

more products available from...
YMAA Publication Center, Inc. 楊氏東方文化出版中心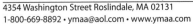

4354 Washington Street Roslindale, MA 02131
1-800-669-8892 • ymaa@aol.com • www.ymaa.com

VIDEOS FROM YMAA

ADVANCED PRACTICAL CHIN NA — 1, 2	T0061, T007X
ARTHRITIS RELIEF — CHINESE QIGONG FOR HEALING & PREVENTION	T558
BACK PAIN RELIEF — CHINESE QIGONG FOR HEALING & PREVENTION	T566
CHINESE QIGONG MASSAGE — SELF	T327
CHINESE QIGONG MASSAGE — PARTNER	T335
COMP. APPLICATIONS OF SHAOLIN CHIN NA 1, 2	T386, T394
EMEI BAGUAZHANG 1, 2, 3	T280, T299, T302
EIGHT SIMPLE QIGONG EXERCISES FOR HEALTH 2ND ED.	T54X
ESSENCE OF TAIJI QIGONG	T238
NORTHERN SHAOLIN SWORD — SAN CAI JIAN & ITS APPLICATIONS	T051
NORTHERN SHAOLIN SWORD — KUN WU JIAN & ITS APPLICATIONS	T06X
NORTHERN SHAOLIN SWORD — QI MEN JIAN & ITS APPLICATIONS	T078
QIGONG: 15 MINUTES TO HEALTH	T140
SHAOLIN KUNG FU BASIC TRAINING — 1, 2	T0045, T0053
SHAOLIN LONG FIST KUNG FU — TWELVE TAN TUI	T159
SHAOLIN LONG FIST KUNG FU — LIEN BU CHUAN	T19X
SHAOLIN LONG FIST KUNG FU — GUNG LI CHUAN	T203
SHAOLIN LONG FIST KUNG FU — YI LU MEI FU & ER LU MAI FU	T256
SHAOLIN LONG FIST KUNG FU — SHI ZI TANG	T264
SHAOLIN LONG FIST KUNG FU — XIAO HU YAN	T604
SHAOLIN WHITE CRANE GONG FU — BASIC TRAINING 1, 2, 3	T440, T459, T0185
SIMPLIFIED TAI CHI CHUAN — 24 & 48	T329
SUN STYLE TAIJIQUAN	T469
TAI CHI CHUAN & APPLICATIONS — 24 & 48	T485
TAI CHI FIGHTING SET	T0363
TAIJI BALL QIGONG — 1, 2, 3, 4	T475, T483, T0096, T010X
TAIJI CHIN NA IN DEPTH — 1, 2, 3, 4	T0282, T0290, T0304, T031
TAIJI PUSHING HANDS — 1, 2, 3, 4	T505, T513, T0134, T0142
TAIJI SABER	T491
TAIJI & SHAOLIN STAFF — FUNDAMENTAL TRAINING — 1, 2	T0088, T0347
TAIJI SWORD, CLASSICAL YANG STYLE	T817
TAIJI WRESTLING — 1, 2	T037, T038X
TAIJI YIN & YANG SYMBOL STICKING HANDS–YANG TAIJI TRAINING	T580
TAIJI YIN & YANG SYMBOL STICKING HANDS–YIN TAIJI TRAINING	T0177
TAIJIQUAN, CLASSICAL YANG STYLE	T752
WHITE CRANE HARD QIGONG	T612
WHITE CRANE SOFT QIGONG	T620
WILD GOOSE QIGONG	T949
WU STYLE TAIJIQUAN	T477
XINGYIQUAN — 12 ANIMAL FORM	T310

DVDS FROM YMAA

ANALYSIS OF SHAOLIN CHIN NA	D0231
BAGUAZHANG 1, 2, 3 — EMEI BAGUAZHANG	D0649
CHEN TAIJIQUAN	D0819
CHIN NA IN DEPTH COURSES 1 — 4	D602
CHIN NA IN DEPTH COURSES 5 — 8	D610
CHIN NA IN DEPTH COURSES 9 — 12	D629
EIGHT SIMPLE QIGONG EXERCISES FOR HEALTH	D0037
THE ESSENCE OF TAIJI QIGONG	D0215
QIGONG MASSAGE—FUNDAMENTAL TECHNIQUES FOR HEALTH AND RELAXATION	D0592
SHAOLIN KUNG FU FUNDAMENTAL TRAINING 1&2	D0436
SHAOLIN LONG FIST KUNG FU — BASIC SEQUENCES	D661
SHAOLIN WHITE CRANE GONG FU BASIC TRAINING 1&2	D599
SIMPLIFIED TAI CHI CHUAN	D0630
SUNRISE TAI CHI	D0274
TAI CHI CONNECTIONS	D0444
TAI CHI ENERGY PATTERNS	D0525
TAI CHI FIGHTING SET—TWO PERSON MATCHING SET	D0509
TAIJI BALL QIGONG COURSES 1&2—16 CIRCLING AND 16 ROTATING PATTERNS	D0517
TAIJI PUSHING HANDS 1&2—YANG STYLE SINGLE AND DOUBLE PUSHING HANDS	D0495
TAIJI PUSHING HANDS 3&4—YANG STYLE SINGLE AND DOUBLE PUSHING HANDS	D0681
TAIJIQUAN CLASSICAL YANG STYLE	D645
TAIJI SWORD, CLASSICAL YANG STYLE	D0452
UNDERSTANDING QIGONG 1	D069X
UNDERSTANDING QIGONG 2	D0418
UNDERSTANDING QIGONG 3—EMBRYONIC BREATHING	D0555
UNDERSTANDING QIGONG 4—FOUR SEASONS QIGONG	D0562
WHITE CRANE HARD & SOFT QIGONG	D637

more products available from...
YMAA Publication Center, Inc. 楊氏東方文化出版中心
4354 Washington Street Roslindale, MA 02131
1-800-669-8892 • ymaa@aol.com • www.ymaa.com